HAYFA BERGAOUI
IMEN GHADHAB
HOUDA MHABRECH

INFILTRATING LOBULAR CARCINOMA OF THE BREAST

HAYFA BERGAOUI
IMEN GHADHAB
HOUDA MHABRECH

INFILTRATING LOBULAR CARCINOMA OF THE BREAST

ScienciaScripts

Imprint

Cover image: www.ingimage.com

This book is a translation from the original published under ISBN 978-620-6-69678-0.

Publisher:
Sciencia Scripts
is a trademark of
Dodo Books Indian Ocean Ltd. and OmniScriptum S.R.L publishing group

120 High Road, East Finchley, London, N2 9ED, United Kingdom
Str. Armeneasca 28/1, office 1, Chisinau MD-2012, Republic of Moldova, Europe
Printed at: see last page
ISBN: 978-620-8-08185-0

Contents

1 INTRODUCTION 2
2 PATIENTS AND METHODS 3
3 RESULTS 6
4 DISCUSSION 29
5 CONCLUSION 53
6 REFERENCES 56
7 APPENDICES 64

1 INTRODUCTION

Invasive lobular carcinoma accounts for 5-15% of breast cancers [1-2], and is now classed as the second most common histological type, after non-specific invasive cancer (NIC).

Its incidence is rising sharply, from 9.5% in 1987 to 15.6% in 1999 (in the United States). [3]

In fact, several studies have concluded that this increase seems to be linked to the frequency of use of hormone replacement therapy after the menopause, which could multiply the risk of developing this condition by a factor of 2 to 3 and to a much greater extent than for non-specific infiltrating carcinoma [4] . Oral contraception and alcohol consumption may also increase the risk of lobular cancer [5-6].

Its specificity lies, on the one hand, in the difficulty of its clinical and radiological diagnosis and, on the other hand, in its anatomopathological aspect and its mode of extension.

Invasive lobular carcinoma is often associated with multifocal and bilateral breast involvement, with metastatic spread that differs from the non-specific type of invasive carcinoma. It metastasises preferentially to the serous membrane and more particularly to the peritoneum.

Patients generally present at a relatively advanced stage at the time of diagnosis.

However, its therapeutic management and prognosis are virtually identical to that of non-specific infiltrating carcinoma.

Given the frequency of hormone receptors in the tumour mass, hormone therapy is an essential part of the therapeutic armoury.

We carried out a retrospective descriptive study based on 30 cases of infiltrating lobular carcinoma of the breast, collected in the Obstetric Gynecology Department of the Maternity and Neonatology Centre of Monastir, for which the histological study was carried out in the anatomopathological laboratory of Monastir over a period of 10 years: from 01 January 2008 to 31 December 2017.

The objectives of our work were to :

- Describe the anatomical and clinical features.
- To clarify the role of breast imaging in the positive diagnosis of invasive lobular carcinoma.
- Describe its therapeutic methods.
- To identify the prognostic factors for invasive lobular carcinoma.

2 PATIENTS AND METHODS

I. Type and population of study

Retrospective descriptive study of 30 observations of CLI of the breast collected in the Obstetric Gynecology Department of the Maternity and Neonatology Centre of Monastir over a 10-year period from 01 January 2008 to 31 December 2017.

II. STUDY POPULATION Study population

1. Inclusion criteria

We included all patients treated in our department for CLI during the study period.

2. Exclusion criteria:

We excluded breast tumours without histological evidence and patients not managed in our department.

III. Definition of study variables

The variables studied were mainly :

1. Epidemiological characteristics

The general characteristics studied are :

> The patient's age at diagnosis.
> The patient's age at menarche and parity.
> Age at first pregnancy.
> The duration of breastfeeding.
> Taking oral contraception.
> Taking hormone replacement therapy
> Personal and family history of breast cancer.
> Personal history of fibrocystic mastopathy of the breast.
> Consumption of toxic substances (alcohol, tobacco).

2. Clinical characteristics

- Anamnesis: delay and reason for consultation.
- Data from the clinical examination :
- Characteristics of the mammary nodule: location, number, size and mobility.
- The presence of inflammatory signs.
- The presence of axillary adenopathy.
- 1 examination of the contralateral breast.
- General physical examination.

3. Radiological diagnostic criteria for breast cancer

Echomammography data is analysed in accordance with the recommendations of the 5eme ACR edition of BIRADS (**Appendix 1**).

3.1. Mammography

> The shape.

> The size.
> Tumour outlines.
> The number of lesions.
> The presence of microcalcifications.
> Other associated lesions (architectural distortion, skin signs, etc.).
> Ganglion areas.

3.2. Breast ultrasound

> The shape.
> Long axis of the mass.
> The size.
> Tumour outlines.
> Subsequent attenuation of echoes.
> Other associated lesions (architectural distortion, skin signs, etc.).
> The number of lesions.
> Ganglion areas.

3.3. Breast MRI

> for examination of the contralateral breast

4. Histological criteria of the tumour diagnosed (Appendix 2)

4.1. Collection methods

> Echo guided biopsy.
> Surgical biopsy.

4.2. Histological criteria

The criteria studied are mainly those necessary to establish the patient's prognosis:

- The number of lesions.
- Multifocal disease.
- Histological tumour size.
- SBR tumour grade.
- The presence of lymph node involvement.
- The status of hormone receptors (R0: restrogen receptor, RP: progesterone receptor).
- HER-2 receptor status; Ki 67.

IV. Therapeutic management

Therapeutic management was discussed at the weekly multidisciplinary staff meetings, which brought together different specialities (gynaecology; radiology; carcinology; anatomopathology).

> Surgical treatment: radical/conservative/remedial.
> Radiotherapy
> chemotherapy

- hormone therapy.
- Targeted therapy.

V. Data collection

The data were collected using medical records, radiological and anatomopathological reports from patients, and follow-up at gynaecology and carcinology outpatient clinics, transcribed onto a pre-established computerised form (**Appendix 3**).

VI. Statistical methodology

The data collected were qualitative in nature, and a descriptive analysis of the sociodemographic, clinical, radiological, anatomical-pathological, therapeutic and prognostic characteristics of the study participants was carried out. The data were entered and processed using SPSS software.

3 RESULTS

I. Epidemiological study

1. Incidence

Over a period of 10 years, from 01 January 2008 to 31 December 2017, 750 women were admitted to the Obstetric Gynecology Department of the Monastir Maternity and Neonatology Centre for treatment of breast cancer, all histological types combined. Of these, 30 had CLI of the breast, a frequency of 4% (Figure 1). We also observed that the incidence of CLI is clearly increasing, rising from 2% in 2008 to 7% in 2017 (Figure 2).

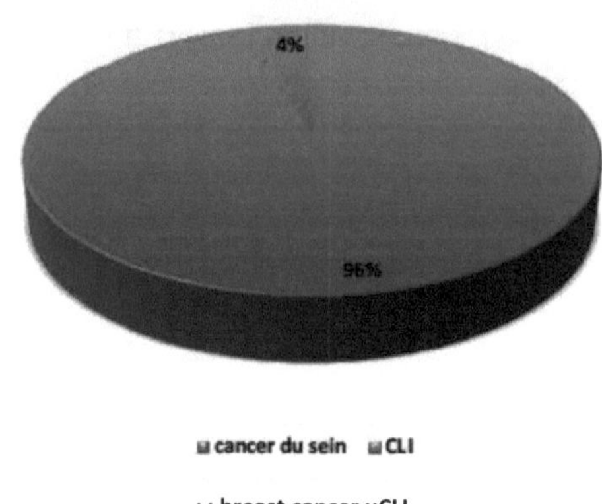

ы breast cancer uCLI

Figure 1: Incidence of CLI during the study period.

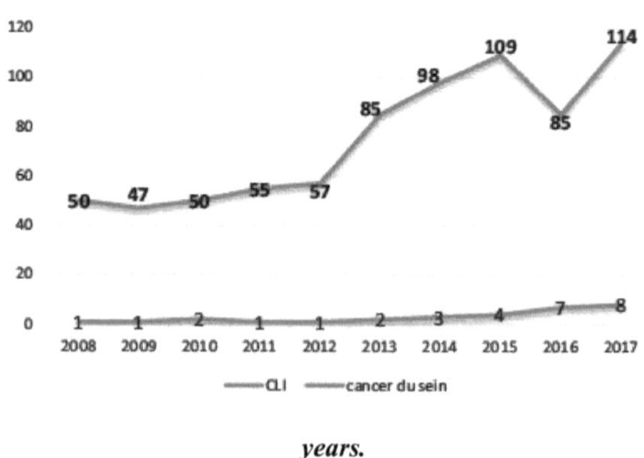

years.

2. Age

The average age of our patients was 53.43 years. The age group most affected was between 50 and 60, representing 40% of cases treated (Figure 3).

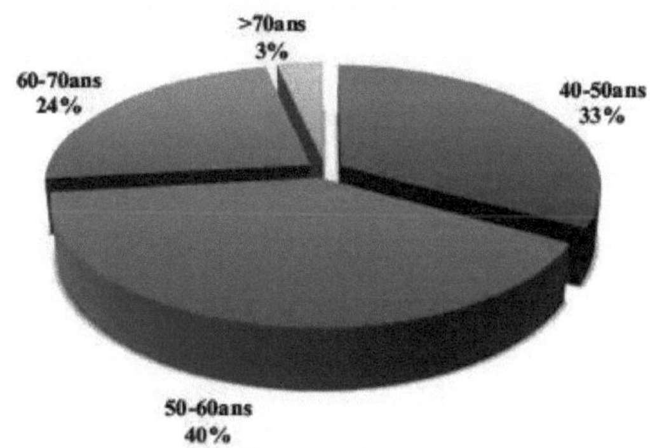

Figure 3: Distribution of patients according to age.

3. Parite

In our series, multiparous women predominated (27 cases), i.e. a frequency of 90%, whereas nulliparous women represented only 3 cases (10%) (Figure 4).

NULLIPARES;

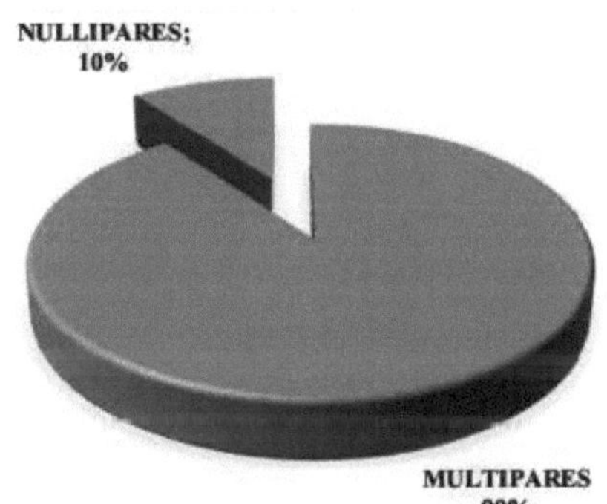

MULTIPARAL 90%

Figure 4: Distribution of patients according to parity.

4. Oral contraception

In our series, 10 women had taken oral contraceptives (33.33% of cases). Thirteen cases had not taken any oral contraceptives (43.33% of cases), while in 7 women (23.33%) the notion of taking contraceptives was not specified (Figure 5).

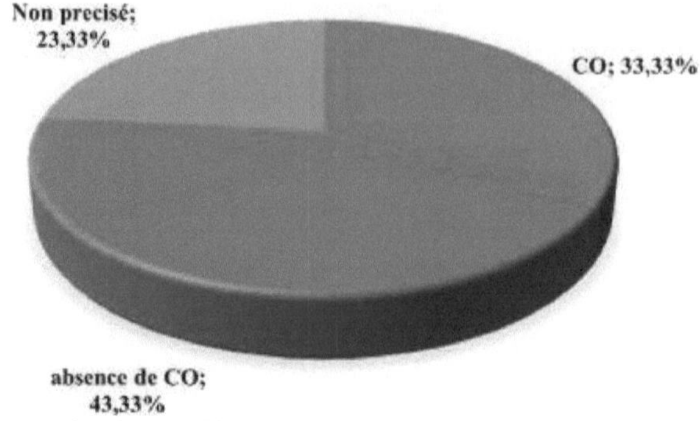

Figure 5: Breakdown of patients taking oral contraceptives

5. Hormonal status

In our series, 16 patients (53.33%) were menopausal (Figure 6).
The age at menopause ranged from 42 to 54 years, with an average of 46.9 years.
The average period of genital activity in this group of women was 37.5 years, with extremes ranging from 28 to 42 years.

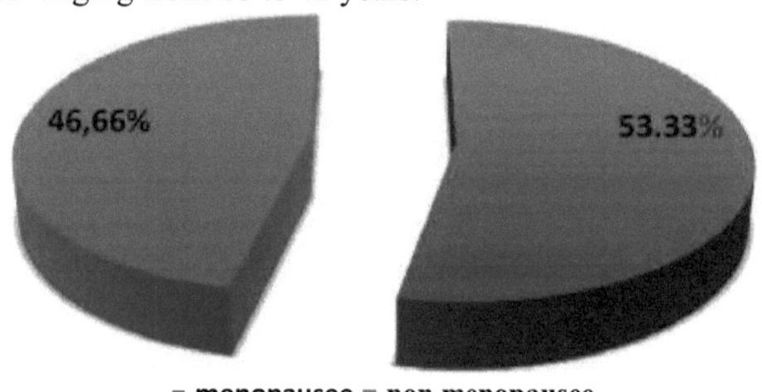

Figure 6: Distribution of patients according to hormonal status.

6. Breastfeeding

Twenty-three cases (76.66%) had breastfed.

7. Background

7.1. Familial breast cancer

Two patients (6.66%) had a family history of breast cancer.

7.2. Employees

History of benign mastopathy was mentioned in only 3 patients (10%).
Only one patient had a personal history of thyroid cancer.

II. Clinical study

1. Consultation deadline

The delay between the appearance of the first signs and the date of consultation was late in the majority of patients. Sixty per cent of patients consulted after 6 months (Figure 7).

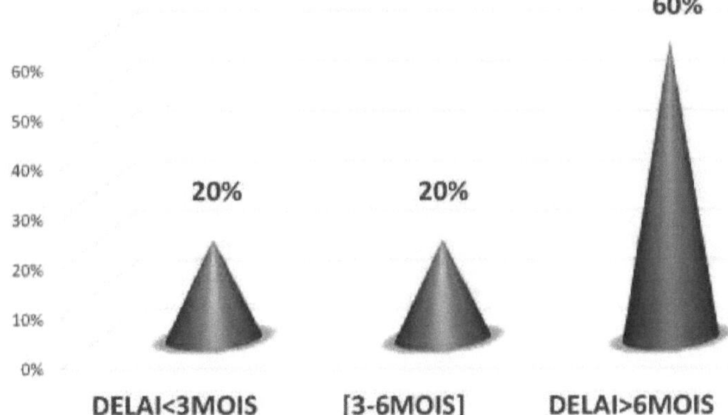

Figure 7: Breakdown of cases according to consultation time.

2. Revealing symptoms

The breast nodule is the most frequent reason for consultation in our series. It represented 83.33% of all symptoms. The most common symptoms, in descending order, were (Figure 8):

A nodule: in 26 cases (83.33%).

Mastodynia: in 5 cases (16.66%).

Screening: in 3 patients (10%).

Breast discharge: in only one patient (3.33%).

Skin redness was observed in only one patient (3.33%).

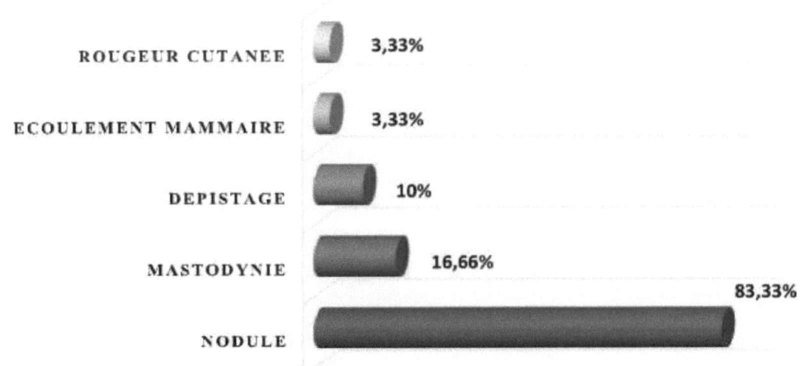

Figure 8: Signs of CLI in our series.

3. Clinical examination

On clinical examination, the presence of :

Nodules: 36 nodules were observed in 29 patients (97%). (Figure 9).

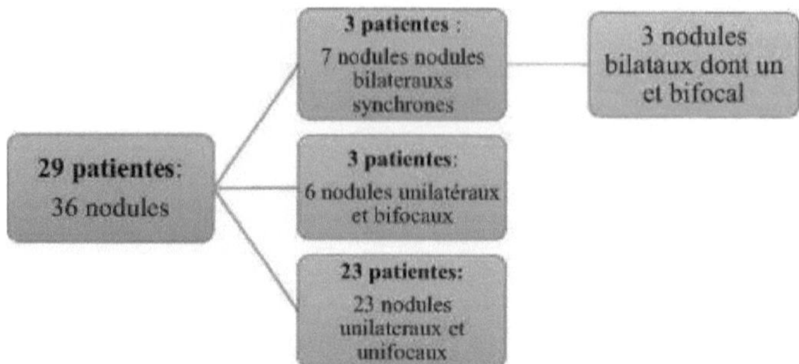

Figure 9: Number of nodules detected on clinical examination.

Breast retraction: was observed in 5 patients (16.66%).
Asymmetry of height: was noted in 3 patients (10%).
Voiding: was found in only one patient (3.33%).
Skin redness: was observed in only one patient (3.33%).
Nipple discharge: was found in only one patient (3.33%).

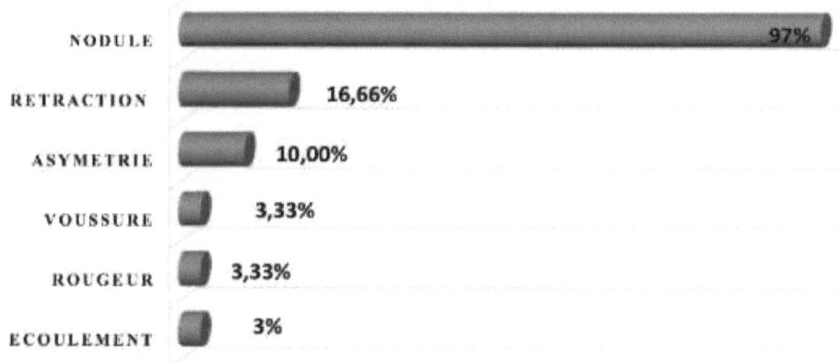

Figure 10: Clinical signs suggestive of CLI in our series.

3.1. Seat

All patients underwent a thorough clinical examination to identify the various clinical features of the nodule.

The tumour was located preferentially in the left breast in 18 patients (62%), in the right breast in 8 patients (27.65%) and bilaterally in 3 patients (10.35%) (Figure 11).

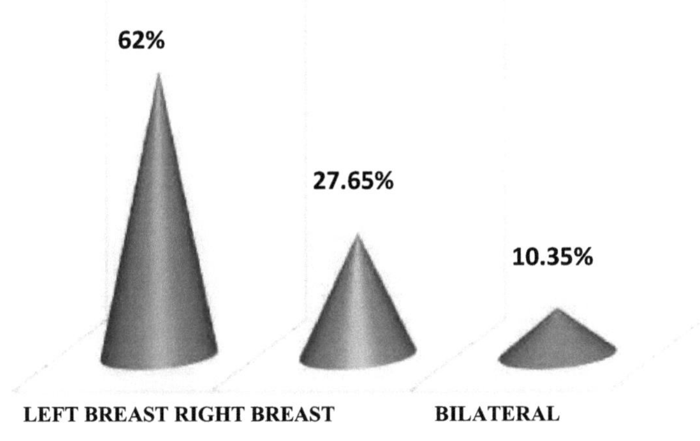

Figure 11: Distribution of patients according to tumour site.

3.2. Topography of the mass

Twenty-one nodules were located in the left breast, of which 9 (42.85%) occupied the superolateral quadrant, and only 8 nodules in the right breast, of which 6 (75%) occupied the right superolateral quadrant (Table I).

Table I: Topography of the nodule in our series.

	QSE	QSI	QII	QIE	JQS	JQI	JQE	JQI	Retromammary
Breast left	9 (42.85%)	3 (14.28%)	1 (4.76%)	3 (14.28%)	1 (4.76%)	2 (9.5%)	1 (4.76%)	0	1 (4.76%)
Right breast	6 (75%)	0	0	0	1 (12.5%)	0	1 (12.5%)	0	0

3.3. Bilaterality

Three patients had synchronous bilateral nodules, one of which was bifocal, giving a total of 7 nodules. (Table II).

Table II: Topography of the nodule in the 3 cases of bilateral CLI

	QSE	QSI	QII	QIE	JQS	JQI	JQE	JQI	Retromamelon
Left breast	2	1	0	0	0	0	0	0	1
Breast right	3	0	0	0	0	0	0	0	0

3.4. Nodule size

At the time of clinical examination, the majority of nodules were larger than 2cm: 22 nodules (61%), distributed as follows (Figure 12):

> 18 nodules, i.e. 50% between 2 and 5 cm.

> 4 nodules, i.e. 11% >5cm in size.

14 nodules (39%) were < 2cm.

The mean tumour size in our series was 3.31 cm, with extremes ranging from 0.8 cm to 9 cm.

11%

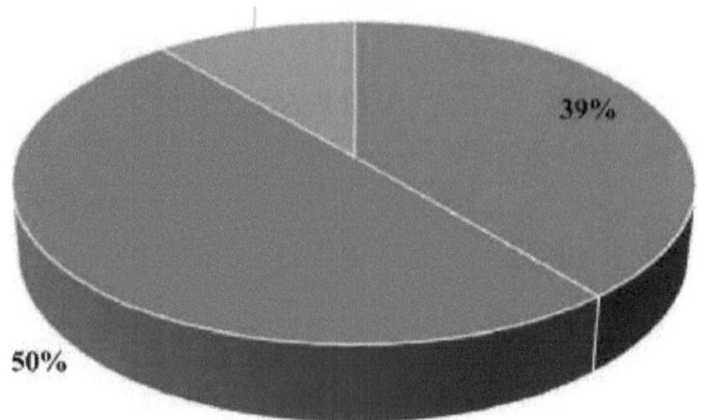

■ size<2cm ■ size(2-5cm) ■ size>5cm

Figure 12: Distribution of patients according to tumour size.

3.5. Other clinical signs

In our series, inflammatory signs were observed in one patient, while 5 patients showed nipple retraction. A tumour extending deep into the skin was found in 02 patients. Superficial (cutaneous) attachment was noted in 03 patients.

3.6. Examination of lymph nodes

Palpation of the lymph nodes revealed homolateral mobile axillary adenopathy in 08 patients (26.66%).

III. Paraclinical study

1. Mammography

Mammography was performed on all our patients and showed: (Figure 13)

1.1. A mass in 29 patients (96.66%).

1.2. Microcalcifications in 8 patients (26.66%).

1.3. Architectural disorganisation in 7 patients (23.33%).

1.4. Skin signs in 7 patients (23.33%).

1.5. Macrocalcifications in 2 cases (6.66%).

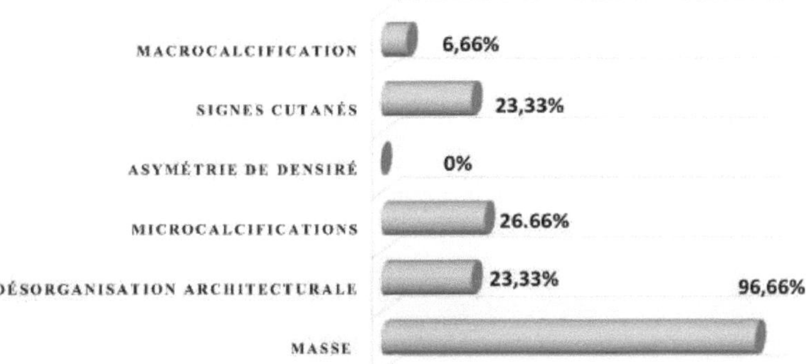

Figure 13: Mammographic aspects of CLI

1.6. Mass

A breast mass was identified in 29 patients.

1.6.1. The number

The total number of masses detected on mammography was 39.

- Unilateral: 26 patients had unilateral masses on mammography. This mass was unifocal in 21 patients (72.41%) and bifocal in 5 patients (17.24%),
- Bilateral: 3 patients had bilateral masses on mammography (10.35%). The mass was multifocal in 2 of these 3 patients, giving a total of 8 masses.

1.6.2. Shape

The mass was :

Round in 2 cases (5.12%).

Non-geometric in 8 cases (20.51%).

Stellar in 29 cases (74.35%) (Figure 14)

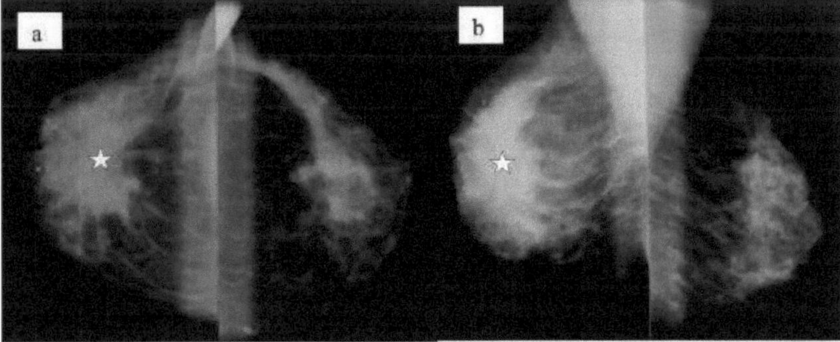

Figure 14: Bilateral mammogram, front view (a) and external oblique view (b): Large, dense, star-shaped mass in the right breast causing asymmetrical density. The left breast is normal. No axillary adenopathy.

1.6.3. Size

The average tumour size on mammography was 2.16 cm, with extremes ranging from 0.5 cm to 5.6 cm.

1.6.4. Contours

The mass was spiculated in 29 cases (74.35%) (Figure 15). It was circumscribed in 2 cases (5.12%) and had indistinct boundaries in 8 cases (20.51%) (Figure 16).

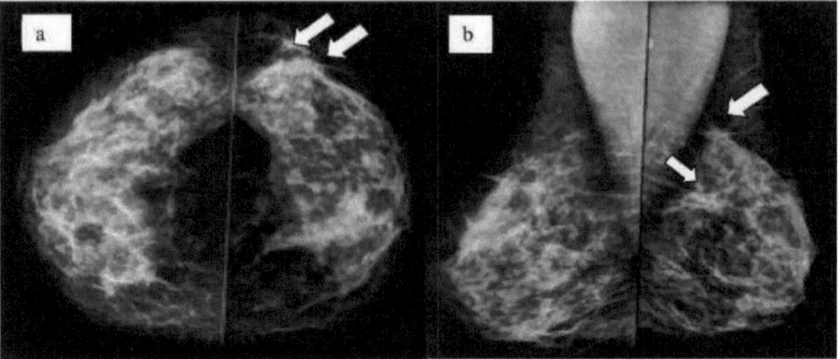

Figure 15: Bilateral mammogram with frontal (a) and external oblique (b) views: breasts of heterogeneous density, BIRADS type "c". 2 masses with stellate outlines located at the level of the QSEG (thick arrows). The right breast is normal in appearance. No axillary adenopathy.

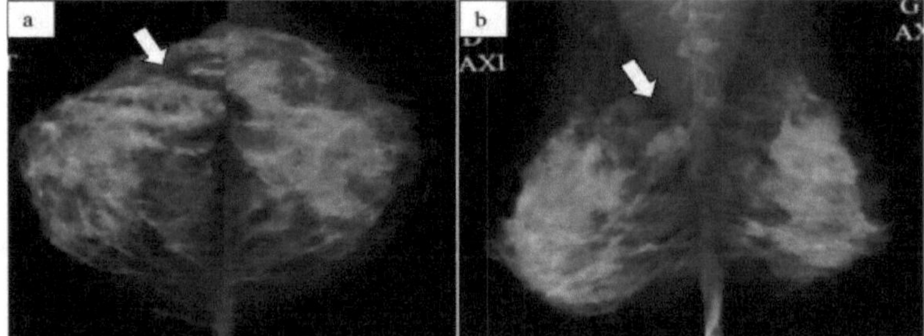

Figure 16: Bilateral mammogram with frontal (a) and external oblique (b) views: breasts of heterogeneous density, BIRADS type "c". A low-density mass, with a mask-like outline in places, is located in the right axillary extension (thick arrow). The left breast is normal. No axillary adenopathy.

1.7. Architectural distortion

A range of architectural disorganisation was observed in 7 patients (23.33%) (Figure 17, 18).

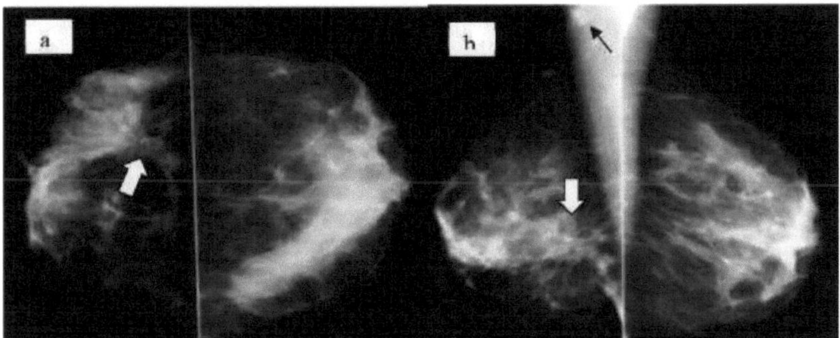

Figure 17: Bilateral mammogram with frontal (a) and external oblique (b) views: BIRADS "c" heterogeneous breast density. Architectural disorganisation of the right QIE (thick arrow). No abnormalities in the left breast. Right axillary ADP (arrow).

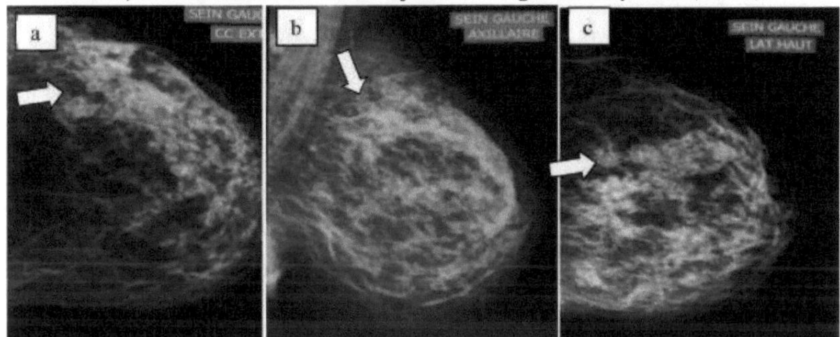

Figure 18: Left unilateral mammogram, front (a), external oblique (b), profile (c): BIRADS "c" heterogeneous breast. Architectural disorganisation of the left QSE (thick arrow). Right axillary ADP (white arrow).

1.8. Microcalcifications

Microcalcifications were observed in 8 patients (26.66%). They were grouped as focal in 3 cases, amorphous in 3 cases and dusty in 2 cases (Figure 19).

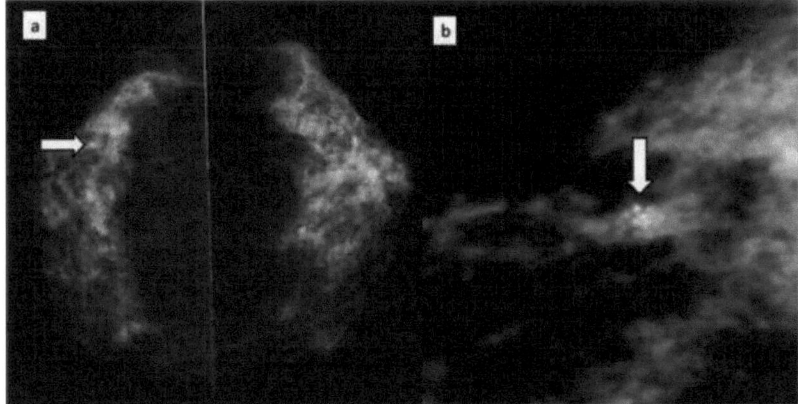

Figure 19: Bilateral mammogram with frontal view (a) and zoom on the right QSE (b):

BIRADS "c" heterogeneous breast density. Focus of amorphous microcalcifications (thick arrow) in the right QSE.

1.9. Associated signs

- Skin signs: skin signs such as skin retraction, skin thickening and nipple retraction were observed respectively in one patient (3.33%), 4 patients (13.33%) and two patients (6.66%) (Figure 20).

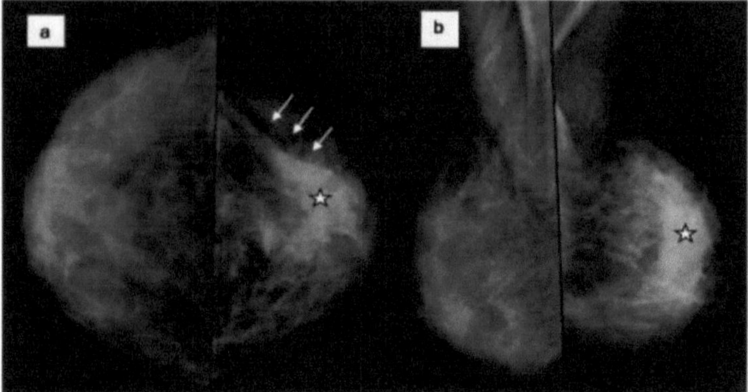

Figure 20: Bilateral mammogram with frontal (a) and external oblique (b) views: asymmetrical breast size with a smaller left breast. This is the site of a dense mass (star) of ill-defined shape and contours, occupying the left breast and accompanied by skin retraction (arrows). The right breast is normal in appearance. No axillary adenopathy.

- Macrocalcifications: images of macrocalcifications were seen in two patients (6.66%).

1.10. Bilaterality

Bilaterality was observed in 3 patients, giving a total of 8 mammographic masses (2 patients had both bilateral and multifocal CLI):

-a single mass with a round shape and circumscribed contours.

- 7 masses were stellar in shape and spiky in outline.

1.11. Ganglion areas

Axillary adenopathy was present in 16 patients (53.33%), two of whom had bilateral axillary PDAs.

2. Breast ultrasound

Breast ultrasound was performed in all patients.

2.1. Mass

A mass was identified in 29 patients.

2.1.1. Number of lesions

The total number of lesions identified was 39 masses. The mass was unifocal in 21 patients (72.41%), bifocal in 5 patients (17.24%), and bilaterally synchronous in 3 patients (10.35%), two of whom had multifocal lesions.

2.1.2. Lesion sites

CLI was most prevalent in the left breast (62%). Twenty-seven percent of the masses were located in the right breast. The mass was located in the left superolateral quadrant in 42.85% of cases.

2.1.3. Size

The average size was 2.36 cm with extremes between 0.6 cm and 6 cm.

2.1.4. Shape

Among the 39 masses :

- Twenty-nine had irregular contours (74.35%).
- Two masses were round (5.12%).
- Eight masses were non-geometric (20.51%) (Figure 21).

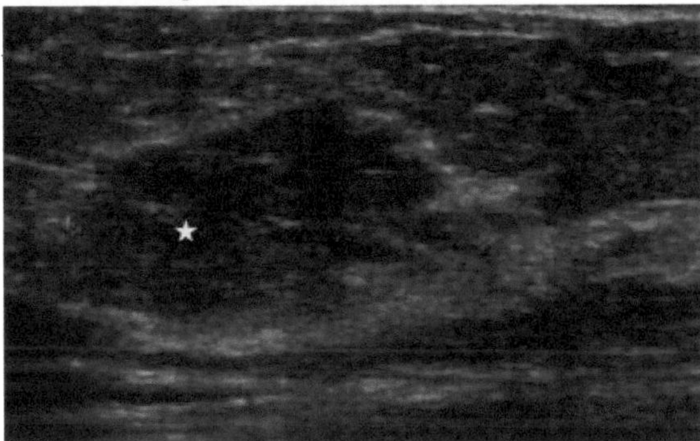

Figure 21: Mammary ultrasound: A heterogeneous hypoechogenic mass (star) with a long axis parallel to the skin, unaccompanied by any changes in the echoes from above. Its contours are irregular.

2.1.5. Tumour contours

Among the 39 masses :

Six were microlobulated (15.38%).

Eight were non-geometric (20.51%).

Ten masks in 10 cases (25.64%).

Fifteen had indistinct contours (38.46%).

In general, the mass was hypoechoic with an uncircumscribed contour in 33 cases (84.61%) and circumscribed in only 6 cases (15.36%).

2.1.6. The main axis of the mass

The long axis of the mass was perpendicular to the skin in 5 cases and parallel to the skin in 7 cases.

2.1.7. Acoustic behaviour

Posterior attenuation of the echoes was observed in 51.72% of cases, and a strengthening of the echoes was visible in 34.48% of cases (Figure 22).

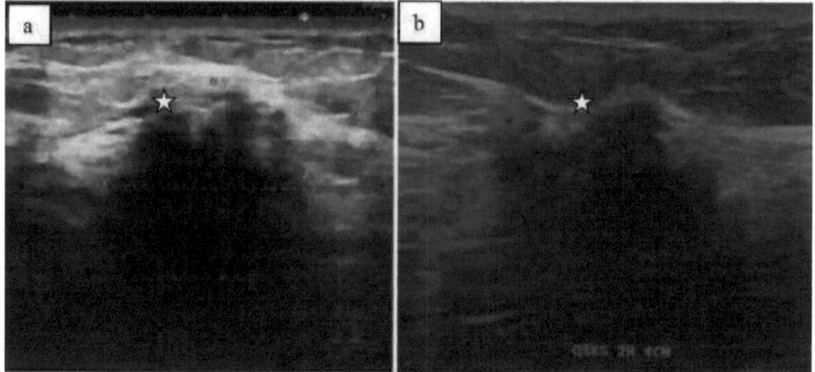

Figure 22: Breast ultrasound (a, b): A hypoechogenic mass (star) with a long axis perpendicular to the skin, accompanied by attenuation of the echoes in the breast.

2.1.8. Echogenic halo around the mass

A hyperechogenic halo was present in 12 cases (30.76%).

2.2. Architectural distortion

Areas of distortion of the breast architecture were observed in 7 patients (23.33%).

2.3. Other associated lesions

- Skin signs: Ultrasound did not identify any skin signs in our series.
- Galactophoric ectasia: No image of galactophoric ectasia.
- Benign lesions: Benign lesions were identified on ultrasound as fibrocystic dystrophies in 1 patient (3.33%) and bilateral microcysts in 3 cases (10%).
- Microcalcifications : Microcalcifications were observed in 8 patients (26.66%).

2.4. Ganglion areas

Axillary adenopathy was observed in 16 patients (53.33%).

3. BIRADS ACR classification :

On completion of the echomammographic work-up, the various lesions were identified according to the ACR classification, taking into account their malignant potential.

In our series the lesions were classified ACR5 in 63.33%, ACR 4 in 36.66% of cases.

cases (Figure 23).

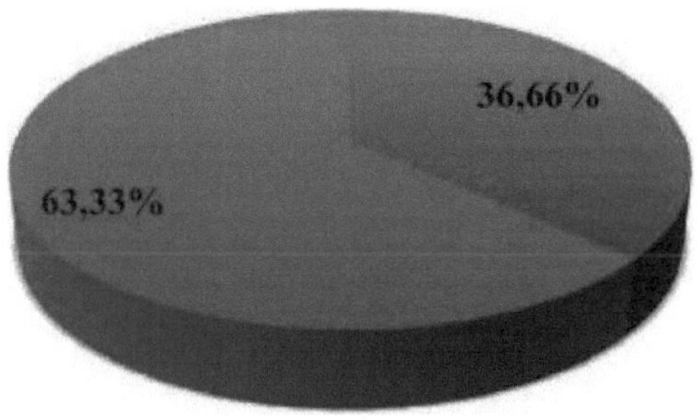

■ ACR4 HACR5

Figure 23: Ultrasound ACR classification

4. Breast MRI

Breast MRI was not part of the initial work-up in our series. It was performed in only 3 patients. In one case, it was performed postoperatively to explore the contralateral breast. In the other two cases, MRI was performed preoperatively to explore a focus of breast dystrophy discovered on ultrasound in one case and to look for multifocal disease in the other.

MRI showed non-mass enhancement in two cases (Figure 24) and bilateral fibrocystic mastopathy in the third.

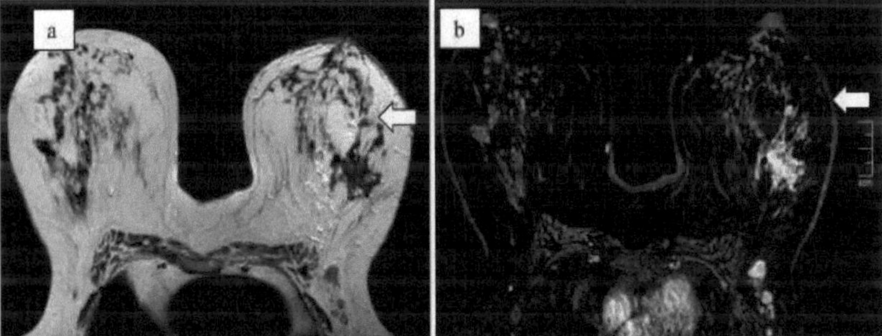

Figure 24: SE T2 (a) and SE T1 axial section breast MRI after dynamic injection of Gadolinium: stellate mass of the left QSE (thick arrow) with non-mass enhancement. Left axillary adenopathy (arrow).

IV. Anatomo-pathological study on biopsy and zonectomy

All suspected radiological masses were biopsied (39 radiological masses) in which the diagnosis of CLI was confirmed. Histological verification by zonectomy after identification of a focus of microcalcifications was carried out in only one patient in whom neither a radiological mass nor a clinical nodule was identified and which showed CLI.

A total of 40 histological results were obtained before surgery, the histological characteristics of which were as follows:

1. Histological type

In 5 cases, CLI was associated with lobular carcinoma in situ (12.5%).

In only one case was CLI associated with CINS (2.5%).

A CLI was found in 34 cases (85%). (Figure 25).

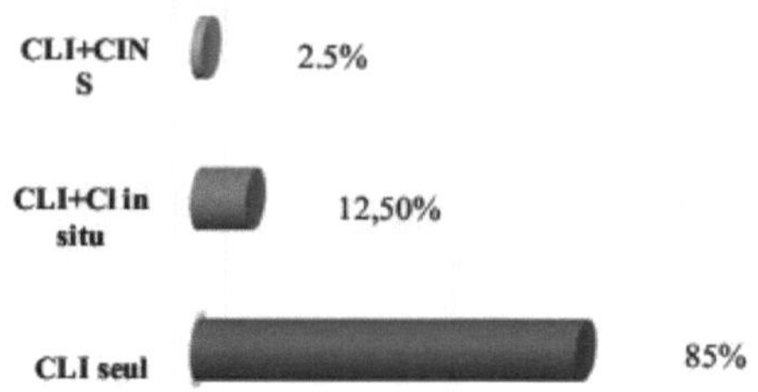

Figure 25: Histological type of tumour

2. Scarf-Bloom and Richardson histo-pronostic grading (SBR)

The SBR grade was specified for all 40 biopsied tumours (Figure 26).

- SBR II for 29 cases, i.e. 72.5%.
- SBR I in 10 cases, i.e. 25%.
- SBR III for a single case, i.e. 2.5%.

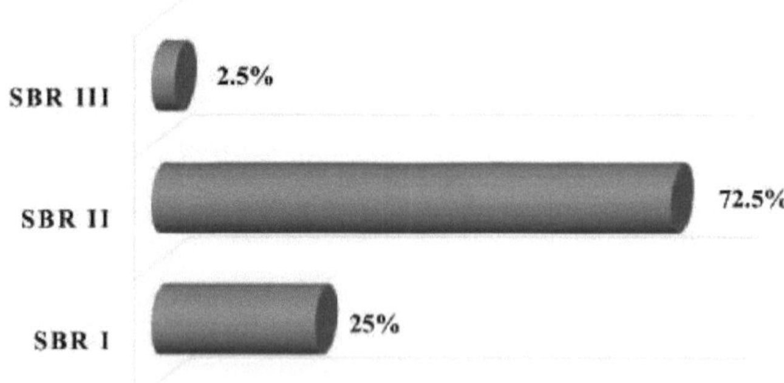

Figure 26: Classification according to SBR grade

3. Immunohistochemical data

3.1. Hormone receptors

Ostrogen and progesterone receptors were detected in all tumour biopsy samples (Figure 27):

38 cases had positive estrogen receptors (95%).

02 cases had negative estrogen receptors (5%).

36 were progesterone receptor positive (90%).

4 did not express progestin receptors (10%)

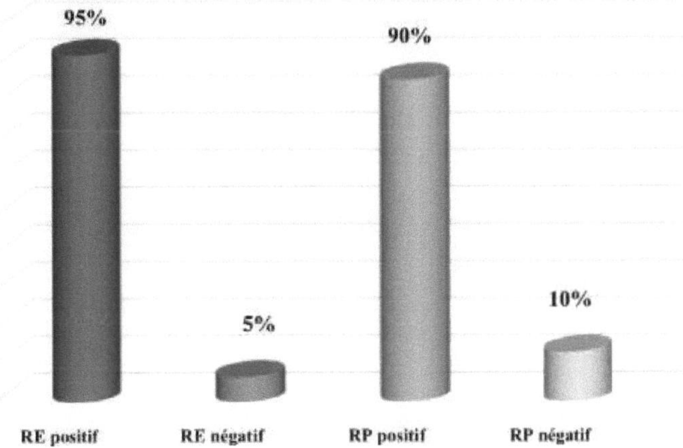

Figure 27: Distribution of estrogen-progestogen receptors.

V. Anatomical-pathological study of the surgical specimen

1. Histological type

The anatomopathological study concerned 31 operative parts from a total of 29 patients operated on (taking into account patients with bilateral CLI: the first patient underwent 2 surgical procedures; radical treatment of the left breast and conservative treatment of the right breast; the second underwent conservative treatment for both breasts and the third was not operated on, making a total of 29 patients operated on from the 30 and 31 operative parts).

- In the 2 patients operated on with bilateral involvement: both patients had bilateral CLI.
- In the remaining 27 operated patients with unilateral involvement, CLI associated with lobular carcinoma in situ was found in 5 patients, CLI associated with NSC in 1 case and CLI in 21 patients.

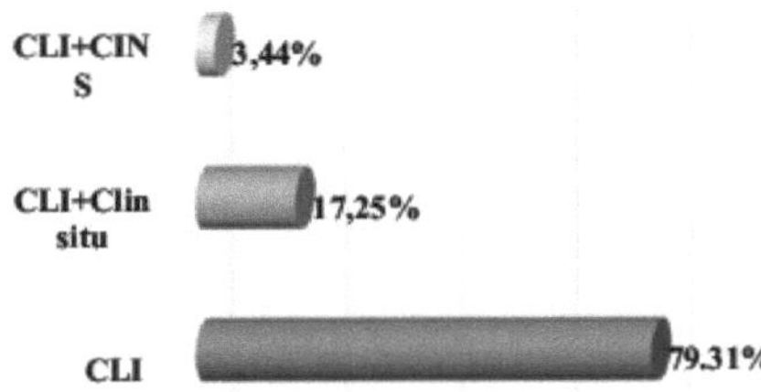

Figure 28: Histological type of tumour

2. Number of lesions

The unifocal feature was found in 17 operating parts from a total of 31. (54.84%).

The bifocal and multifocal characteristics were found in 6 and 8 cases respectively, i.e. a percentage of 19.36% and 25.80%. (Figure 29).

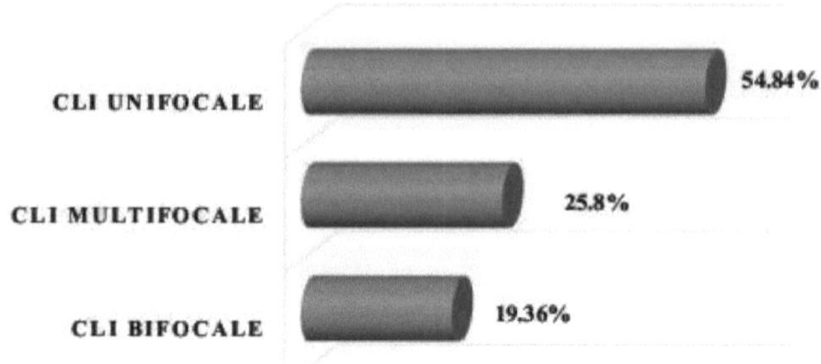

Figure 29: Breakdown of CLI by number of households

3. Histological lymph node involvement

Lymph node dissection was positive in 21 patients (72.41%).

The number of lymph nodes affected is detailed in the figure below. (Figure 30)

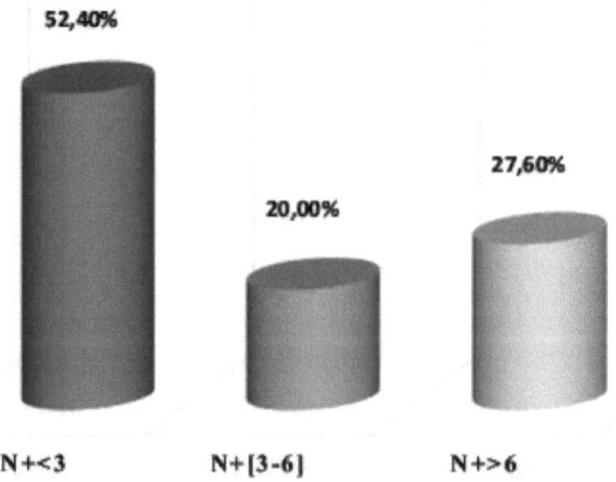

Figure 30: Number of lymph nodes affected

4. Capsular rupture

Two cases of capsular rupture were identified on pathological examination (6.45%).

5. Tumour size

The average tumour size was 3.27 cm, with extremes ranging from 1 cm to 6.5 cm.

6. Vascular emboli

No cases of vascular emboli were found in our series.

7. Scarf-Bloom and Richardson histo-pronostic grading (SBR)

The SBR grade was specified for all 31 surgical parts (Figure 31).
SBR II for 23 cases, i.e. 74.2%.
SBR I in 7 cases, i.e. 22.58%.
SBR III for a single case, i.e. 3.22%.

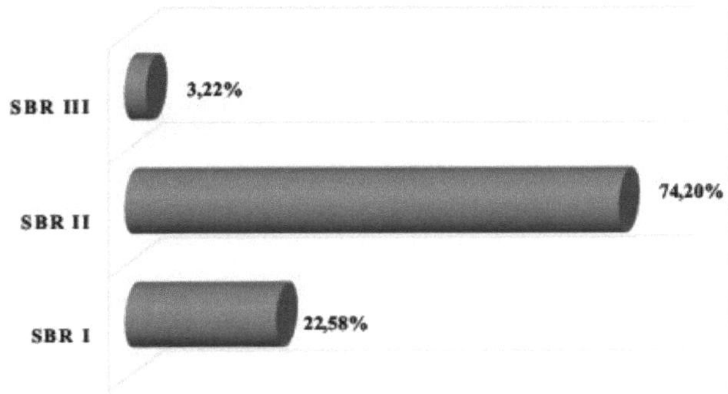

Figure 31: Classification according to SBR grade

8. Immunohistochemical data

8.1. Hormone receptors

Ostrogenic and progestogen receptors were investigated for all surgical parts (Figure 32):
29 tumours had positive estrogen receptors (93.55%).
02 had negative estrogen receptors (6.45%).
27 were progesterone receptor positive (87.1%).
28 did not express progestin receptors (12.9%).

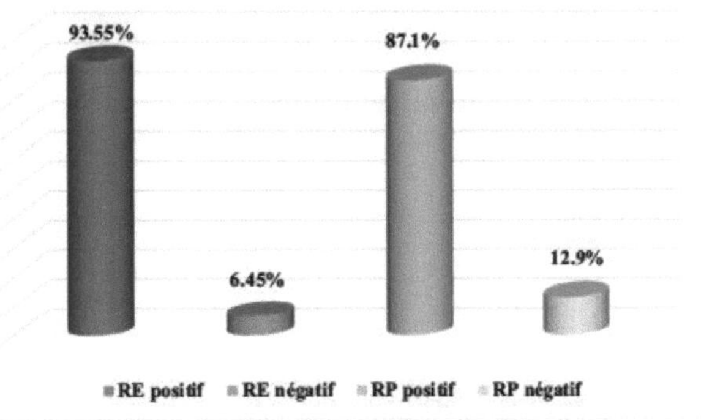

Figure 32: Distribution of estrogen-progestogen receptors.

8.2. HER2 receptors

In our series, the majority of tumours did not express the HER2 receptor (Figure

33).
4 cases (12.9%) expressed the HER-2 receptor.
HER-2 was negative in 27 cases (87.1%).

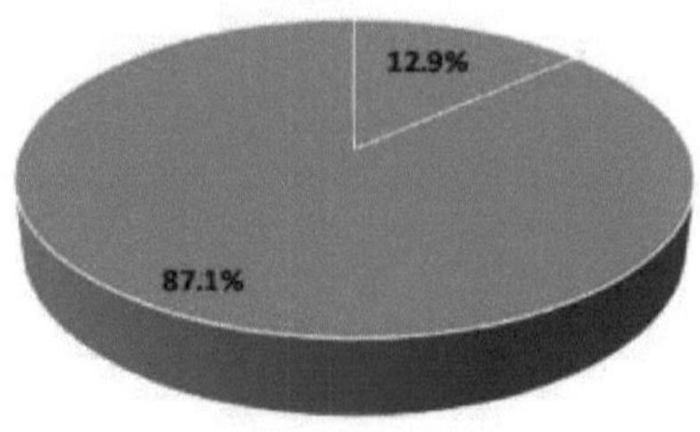

Figure 33: Distribution of patients according to HER2 expression.

8.3. KI 67

The ki67 proliferation factor was greater than 20% in 3 patients.

VI. Assessment of extension

The aim of the extension work-up is to look for secondary locations in order to classify the tumour and determine its initial prognosis. The work-up typically comprises a clinical and paraclinical component.

1. General assessment of extension

1.1. Clinic

A general examination was performed in all patients. No abnormalities were detected in 29 patients, apart from hepatomegaly in one case.

1.2. Clinical Para

1.2.1. Chest X-ray

Chest X-rays were carried out in all patients and did not reveal any abnormalities.

1.2.2. Abdominal and pelvic ultrasound

Abdominal and pelvic ultrasound showed hepatic metastasis in only one case.

1.2.3. Bone scan

It was normal in all patients.

1.2.4. CA 15-3

CA15-3 levels were high (10 times normal) in the patient with hepatic metastasis.

1.2.5. Thoracic, abdominal and pelvic CT

It was performed on a single patient to look for a secondary location.

VII. TNM classification

1. T: tumour size

The 36 nodules found on clinical examination included :

14 nodules were classified as T1 (38.88%).
16 nodules were classified as T2 (44.44%).
2 nodules were classified T3 (5.57%).
4 nodules were classified T4 (11.11%). (Figure 34).

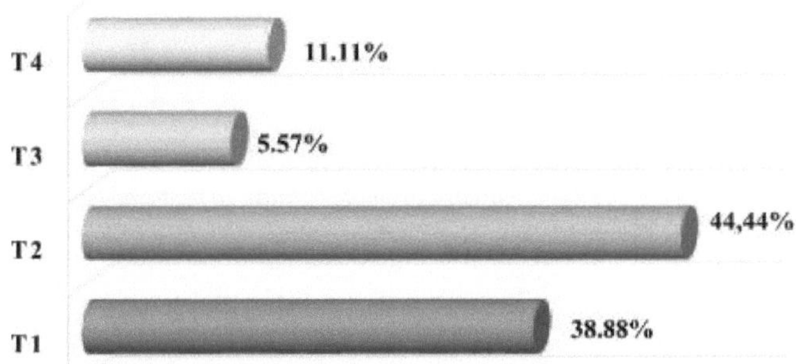

Figure 34: TNM classification according to T size.

2. N: regional adenopathies

The clinical examination revealed the following (Figure 35):
Homolateral mobile adenopathies (N1): 11 cases (36.66%).
Fixed homolateral adenopathies (N2): absent.
Contralateral adenopathies (N3): absent.
Absence of regional adenopathy (N0): 19 cases (63.33%).

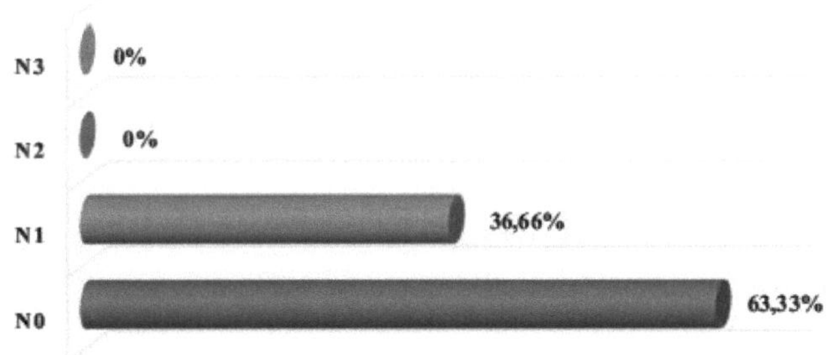

Figure 35: TNM classification according to locoregional adenopathies

3. M: Metastases

Only one patient had a secondary location in the liver at the time of diagnosis (Figure 36).

3,33%
MI

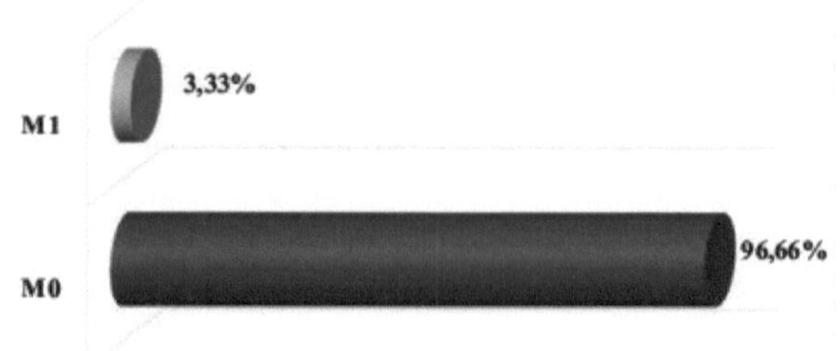

Figure 36: TNM classification according to metastasis

VIII. Therapeutic methods

All cases were discussed at a multidisciplinary consultation meeting (RCP) for a therapeutic decision. A total of 31 surgical procedures were performed, including 2 bilateral CLI in 2 patients.

The total number of patients operated on was 29, as one case of metastatic synchronous bilateral CLI was not operated on. (Figure 37)

1. Surgery

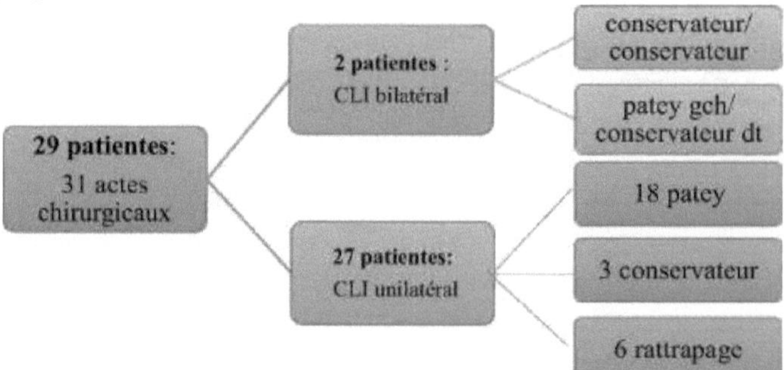

Figure 37: Repair of surgical procedures

1.1. Patey

Taking into account the bilateral nodules, 19 radical surgical procedures of the Patey type were performed, i.e. (61.3%) of a total of 31 surgical procedures.

1.2. Conservative treatment

Six conservative lumpectomy operations with homolateral axillary lymph node dissection (19.35%).

1.3. Catch-up treatment

Salvage mastectomy was indicated in 06 cases because of unhealthy tumour margins, i.e. 19.35% (Figure 38).

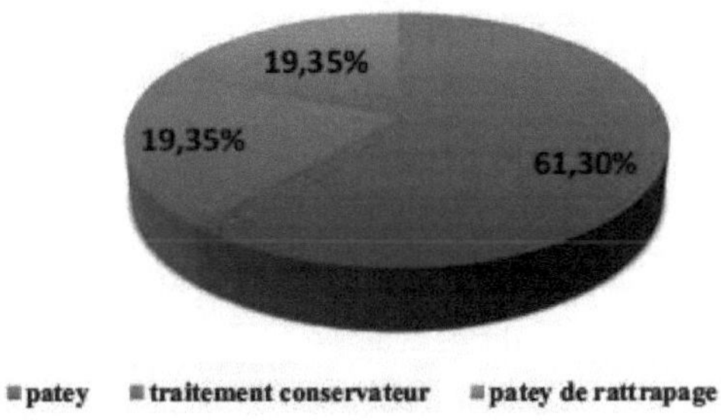

Figure 38: Distribution according to surgical treatment modality.

2. Radiotherapy

External radiotherapy was performed on 28 patients (93.33%): 25 sessions: 2 GY per session every day; 5 days a week; for 5 weeks of treatment.

3. Chemotherapy

3.1. Adjuvant chemotherapy

Twenty-three patients (76.66%) had received adjuvant chemotherapy.

3.2. Neoadjuvant chemotherapy

Neoadjuvant chemotherapy based on PEC100 and docetaxel: 6 courses every 21 days, was indicated in 4 patients (13.33%), with a partial response after chemotherapy, all of whom subsequently underwent radical treatment.

3.3. Palliative chemotherapy

Carried out on a patient with metastatic disease.

4. Hormonotherapy

Adjuvant hormone therapy was performed in 28 patients (93.33%). The protocol differed according to their hormonal status.

4.1. Before the menopause

Hormone therapy with Tamoxifen was indicated in 12 patients (42.85%).

4.2. After the menopause

Hormone therapy with antiaromatase was prescribed in 16 cases (57.15%).

5. Targeted therapy

Herceptin-based targeted therapy was indicated for 4 patients with HER2 overexpression (13.33%).

IX. Evolution

Immediate post-operative follow-up was favourable for all our patients during their hospitalisation. Late complications: there were no local recurrences or distant metastases in all our patients, but 4 cases of lymphoceles were observed.

X. Monitoring

Our operated patients were monitored jointly by an oncologist and a gynaecologist, with a clinical examination every 3 months in the first year and

every 6 months thereafter for 5 years, then once a year for life. This examination covers the 2 breasts, the chest wall and the satellite lymph nodes.
The 1st mammogram was performed 6 months after the end of treatment, and repeated every year thereafter. Surveillance was carried out on the contralateral breast, given the frequency of contralateral cancers in CLI.

XI. Survival

In our series, the 5-year survival rate was 77.3%. (Figure 39)

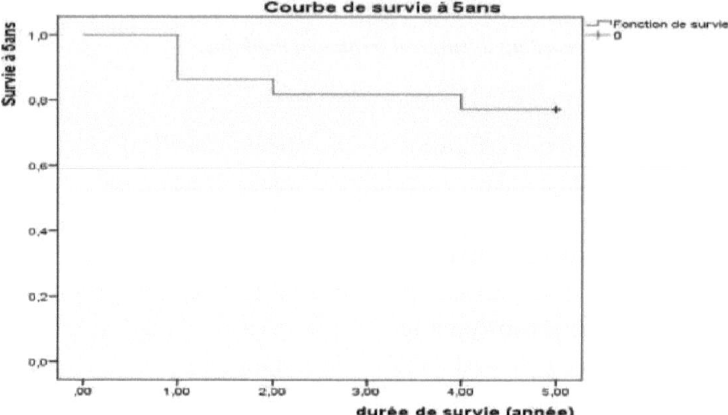

Figure 39: 5-year overall survival curve

4 DISCUSSION

I. Epidemiology

1. Frequency

Breast cancer is currently the leading cancer in women worldwide, dominated by invasive cancer, which accounts for more than 90% of all histological types [4].

Among invasive carcinomas, CLI remains special because of its diagnostic difficulty and its mode of proliferation.

CLI accounts for 5-15% of breast cancers [1; 2]. It is the second most common histological type of breast cancer after NSCLC.

Its incidence is rising sharply, from 9.5% in 1987 to 15.6% in 1999 in the United States. Some hypotheses have attributed this rise to the increase in the prescription of hormone replacement therapy and oral contraception [3].

In Switzerland, a study also showed a 14.4% increase in the frequency of CLI over the period 1976-1999 [7].

This result was also demonstrated in our study, with an increase in the frequency of CLI from 2% in 2008 to 7% in 2017.

In fact, several studies have concluded that this increase seems to be linked to the frequency of use of hormone replacement therapy (HRT) after the menopause, which could multiply the risk of developing CLI by a factor of 2 to 3, and to a much greater extent than for CINS. Alcohol consumption may also increase the risk of lobular cancer, but not all studies agree on this point [5,6].

The evolution and development of diagnostic methods such as ultrasound and MRI, which are more sensitive than mammography in detecting CLI [8], as well as improvements in histopathological techniques, may also contribute to the increase in the detection rate of CLI, explaining its growing incidence in recent years.

The incidence of CLI differs from one population to another (Figure 40):

In the United States, Wasfi et al [9] showed that CLI accounted for 10.5% of all cases of breast cancer.

In South Korea, this frequency is estimated at 2.8% according to Jung et al [10].

In France, Sastre Garau et al [11] found a frequency of 6.5%.

In Tunisia, according to Khlifi et al [12], this frequency was 5.4%.

In our series, the frequency of CLI was estimated at 4%.

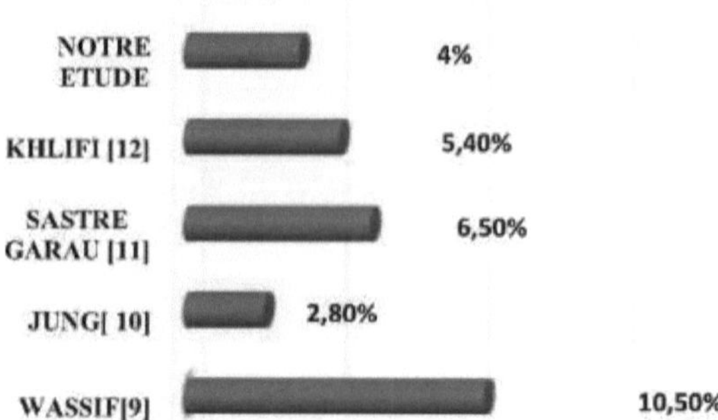

Figure 40: CLI frequency by series.

2. Age

CLI mainly affects older women, often menopausal, and compared with CINS, it occurs in women who are generally 3 years older [13].

The average age varies from one study to another (Figure 41):

For Wasfi et al [9], the mean age was 64.9 years, with extremes ranging from 51 to 78.

According to the study by Jung et al [10], CLI affects women 10 to 20 years younger in the Asian population and the average age at onset of these tumours was 48.4 years.

According to Fortunato et al [14] the average was 63 years.

According to Khlifi et al [12] the average age was 51 years (with extremes ranging from 31 to 86 years).

In our series, the mean age at onset of CLI was 53.43 years, with extremes ranging from 40 to 79 years, and the age group between 40 and 50 years was the most affected.

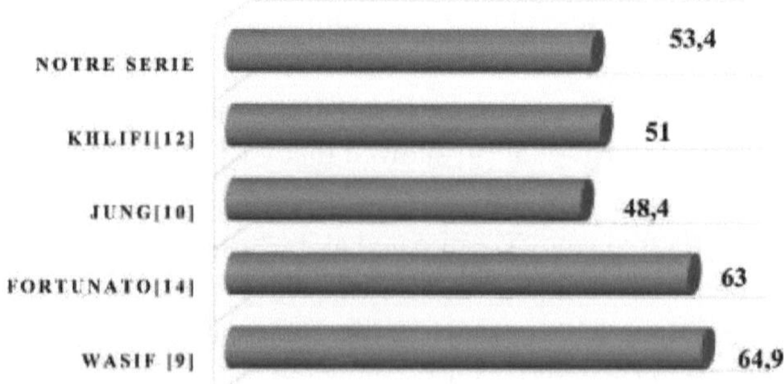

Figure 41: Average age of patients with CLI in different studies.

3. Risk factors

3.1. Menarches

Early onset of breast cancer is considered to be one of the major risk factors for the development of breast cancer. This parameter seems to be slightly more

involved in CLI than in CINS [15].
In our study, the average age of first regies was 12.5 years, with extremes ranging from 11 to 17 years.

3.2. Parity, age at first pregnancy

According to the study by newcomb et al [16], nulliparity and late age at first pregnancy are risk factors for breast CLI.
A late first pregnancy after the age of 30 was associated with a 2.4-fold increase in the risk of CLI compared with a first pregnancy before the age of 20 (OR, 2.4; 95% CI, 1.9-2.9). The association was less pronounced for CINS (OR, 1.3; 95% CI, 1.2-1.4).
Nulliparity was associated with an increased risk for all breast cancer subtypes, compared with women under 20, but the association was stronger with lobular (OR, 1.7; 95% CI, 1.3-2.2) than with ductal (OR, 1.2; 95% CI, 1.1-1.3).
In our series, the results are inconsistent with the literature, as nulliparous women accounted for only 10% of cases, whereas almost all patients who developed CLI were multiparous, but we did not have details of the age of the first pregnancy in all our files.

3.3. Menopause

Late menopause increases the risk of CLI (3.6% increase per year versus 2.6% for CINS) [15].
In our series, 53.33% of patients were menopausal, with an estimated mean age of menopause of 46.9 years, ranging from 42 to 54 years, and an estimated mean age of genital activity of 37.5 years (ranging from 28 to 42 years).

3.4. Breastfeeding

According to Christopher et al [17], breastfeeding does not appear to be a protective factor against CLI, since in their study, compared with women who had never breastfed, those who had breastfed for more than 24 months had a reduced risk of CINS but not for CLI.
In our series, 76.66% of women with CLI breastfed, but the duration of breastfeeding was not mentioned in all the files studied.

3.5. Hormone replacement therapy

Several studies have shown that there is a causal link between hormone replacement therapy and the development of CLI, since it increases the risk of this condition by a factor of 2 to 3, and to a much greater extent than CINS [18].
Reeves et al, found a relative risk for HRT use after the menopause of 2.25 (CI: 2.00-2.52) for lobular cancers and 1.63 (1.551.72) for ductal cancers [19].
In our study, this hypothesis was not supported, as none of our patients had received hormone replacement therapy.

3.6. Personal history of benign mastopathy

Certain benign breast tumours such as fibrocystic mastopathy or lobular hyperplasia, and especially proliferative and atypical mastopathy, increase the risk of breast cancer.

According to the study by Dupont and Pagedans [20] involving 1835 patients, adenofibromas were a risk factor for the development of breast cancer in the long term. These cancers may be of different types: lobular, ductal, infiltrating or "in-situ".

In our series, only 03 patients reported a personal history of benign mastopathy, which represented 10% of all cases studied.

3.7. Family background

Genetic factors certainly play a role and increase the risk of CLI, since they are linked to several mutations, including the CDH1 mutation, which is the most frequent in CLI [21]. This mutation is all the more important when CLI is bilateral and occurs at a young age. Similarly, the BRCA2 mutation on chromosome 13 and the BRCA1 mutation on chromosome 17 increase the incidence of CLI by 8.4% and 2.2% respectively [22].

For Khlifi, [12] 8.1% of patients had a family history of breast cancer, and according to the study by El Alouani, this rate was 14%. [23]

In our series, only one patient (3.33%) had a family history of breast cancer, but a genetic study was not carried out.

3.8. History of lobular carcinoma in situ

This tumour represents 1 to 8% of breast cancers and occurs two times out of three before the menopause. This lesion is considered by some to be a simple factor favouring the development of a subsequent cancer, and by others to be a transitional stage towards the development of an invasive cancer [24].

In our study, none of the patients had antecedents of lobular carcinoma in situ, but at the time of diagnosis we found an association of CLI and CLinsitu in 5 cases.

II. Clinical study

1. Consultation deadline

CLI often evolves in a quiescent manner: a consultation period of over 6 months has been generally demonstrated in several studies: this period was 7.8 months on average for Khlifi [12], and 7 months for El Alouani [23].

In our study, 60% of patients consulted us after 6 months.

2. Reason for consultation

CLI is most often symptomless and usually appears as a fairly large, poorly defined mass that is difficult to distinguish. In some cases, there is only an overall thickening of the mammary gland or a diffuse multi-nodular appearance.

This phenomenon is linked to the fact that CLI is characterised by a less marked or even absent stromal reaction and insidiously infiltrates the mammary gland, which could explain its late diagnosis [25].
Nipple discharge, mastodynia, breast deformity and/or enlargement, nipple retraction or redness of the breast may also be signs of CLI.
According to the study by Cao et al [26], the revealing symptom was a nodule in 84.9%, microcalcifications in 13.2% and nipple discharge in 1.9%.
According to Khlifi [12], the major symptom was a nodule in 87.8% of cases, and similarly for El Alouani, nodules accounted for 80% of the reasons for consultation [23].
In line with the literature, the nodule was the most frequent tell-tale sign in our series with a percentage of 83.33% (Figure 42).

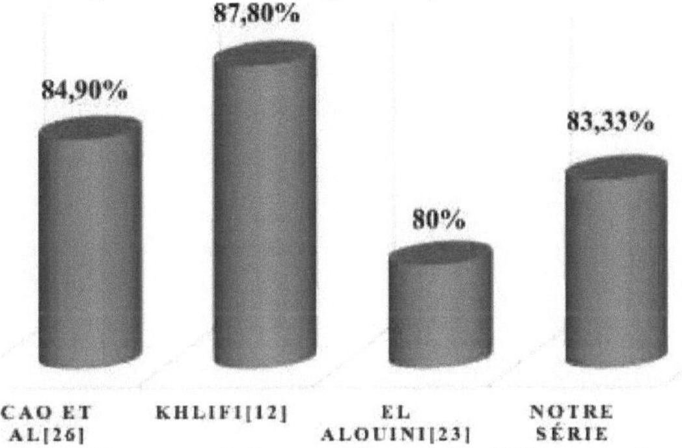

Figure 42: Frequency of breast nodule according to the different series.

3. Physical examination

3.1. Tumour site

According to several studies, CLI is more likely to occur in the left breast. According to Wasfi et al [9], the tumour is found in the left breast in 50.9% of cases.
In our series, according to the literature, 62% of tumours were on the left side.
If we study the tumour in the breast itself, we find that the different quadrants can be affected to varying degrees, but according to several authors, the superolateral quadrant is the most frequently affected:
According to Wasfi et al [9], CLI occurs in the superolateral quadrant in 36.7% of cases. The second most common site is the retromammary area, followed by the superinternal quadrant.
In our series, the tumour was most frequently found in the left superolateral quadrant in 42.85% of cases.

3.2. Multifocalite

One of the particularities of CLI is the multifocal involvement of the mammary parenchyma. In a series of 130 CLI cases, Tot et al found 49% uni-focal involvement, 12% multifocal involvement and 28% diffuse infiltration [27].

According to our study, on clinical examination, 3 patients (10.35%) had bifocal lesions and only one had both multifocal and bilateral lesions (3.44%).

3.3. Bilaterality (figure 43)

One of the major features of CLI is bilateral involvement. This has been demonstrated by several authors who have found a high incidence of bilateral tumours in patients with CLI [28].

Polednak et al [29] carried out a comparative study of 300 cases of bilateral and synchronous breast cancer versus 13,495 patients with unilateral breast cancer, and found that in bilateral forms, CLI was most common.

In a similar study of 143 cases of synchronous bilateral breast cancer, Intra et al [30] also found that CLI was more frequent in bilateral forms (15.5%).

In a retrospective analysis by Goldflam et al [31] of 239 patients with CLI who underwent prophylactic contralateral mastectomy, they found 49 CINS lesions and other moderate or high risk lesions in the contralateral mastectomy specimen at a frequency of 20.5%.

In our study, bilateral tumour involvement was noted in 03 patients, i.e. 10.35% of cases.

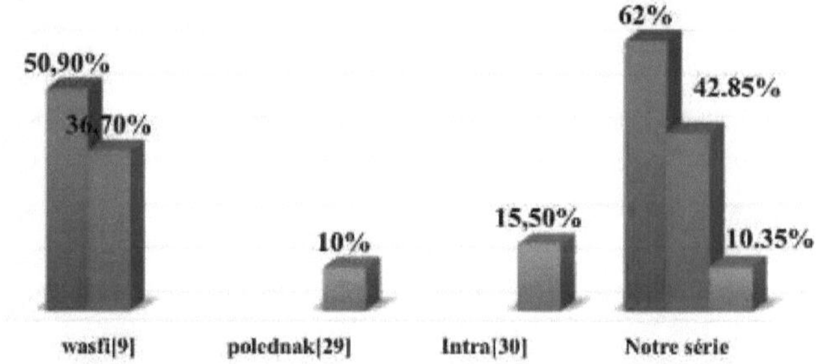

Figure 43: The CLI headquarters in the different series.

3.4. Clinical size

CLI is usually diagnosed at a late stage; in a study by Pestalozzi et al, 55.1% of masses were larger than 2 cm [32].

In our series, the majority of tumours were larger than 2 cm at diagnosis (61%), 11% of which were larger than 5 cm, and the mean tumour size was estimated at 3.31 cm, which is consistent with the literature.

3.5. Limits of the tumour

Clinically, CLI often presents as poorly defined masses with irregular contours [33].

These findings were confirmed in our series, since the mass was poorly limited and had irregular contours in 74.35% of cases.

3.6. Examination of lymph nodes

Patient survival is inversely proportional to lymph node involvement, which is one of the prognostic factors for NSCLC of the breast [34]. The number of lymph nodes affected guides therapeutic management and the choice of adjuvant therapies.

Although CLI is most often diagnosed at an earlier stage than CIN, and despite its large size at diagnosis, it has been observed that the rate of lymph node involvement is the same or even slightly lower than CIN [12].

According to KHLIFI [12] and Alouini [23], homolateral axillary adenopathy was found in 45.9% and 51.66% of cases respectively.

In our study, homolateral mobile axillary adenopathy was found in 36.66% of patients.

III. Medical imaging

The low density of tumour cells and the absence of stromal reaction make CLI difficult to detect by simple physical examination or mammography.

Mammography has a low sensitivity (57-79%) for detecting CLI. This has led to interest in other imaging modalities, such as ultrasound, magnetic resonance imaging, tomosynthesis and targeted molecular imaging [35].

1. Mammography

The ultimate aim of mammography is the early detection of breast cancer. Detailed, high-quality, high-resolution images based on the contrast differences between normal and lesioned breast tissue are the fundamental elements that enable malignant lesions to be detected by mammography.

When these contrast differences are small, detection of breast cancer by mammography becomes increasingly difficult.

CLI infiltrates breast tissue insidiously, spreading in single rows of malignant cells while respecting the underlying anatomical structure. Thus, at an early stage of development and even in advanced stages, CLI can often escape detection by mammography, whose sensitivity for detecting all types of invasive breast carcinoma, including CLI, varies from 63% to 98% [36].

Furthermore, it is well documented that the degree of fibroglandular tissue density is inversely correlated with mammographic sensitivity: when breast tissue is described as heterogeneous or extremely dense, the sensitivity of mammography in detecting invasive tumours also becomes low, at only 30 to 48% [37].

Berg et al specifically examined the performance of mammography as a function of tumour type and breast density. Mammographic sensitivity was 81%

for CINS compared with 34% for CLI. When only patients with dense breast tissue were considered, sensitivity decreased dramatically to 60% and 11%, respectively. [38]

Overall, the most common mammographic findings during CLI are as follows:

1.1. Spicule mass

In the series by Evans et al, a spiculated mass with a dense centre was found in 60% of cases and is classically considered suspicious [39].

Furthermore, Hilleren et al [40] noted that 50% of spiculated CLI masses had a central density less than or equal to that of normal breast parenchyma on all the incidences obtained.

In our study, a spiculated mass was noted in 74.35% of cases.

1.2. Isolated distortion of the architecture

Apart from spiculated masses, one of the most frequent mammographic manifestations in CLI is architectural distortion, which represents around 14 to 25% of the images detected by mammography and is less often associated with microcalcifications [40].

It should be remembered that any glandular asymmetry should prompt the use of centre views with enlargement.

Architectural distortion is identified on mammography when the normal architecture of the breast parenchyma is distorted, but no discernible or discrete mass is evident.

In our series, a range of architectural distortion was observed in 7 patients (23.33%).

1.3. Focal asymmetry of density

A simple asymmetry of density in a dense breast should attract attention. Clinical examination can sometimes reveal an induced mass. In such cases, the centre films may be negative, and only breast ultrasound can reveal a tumour mass. In our series, no cases of asymmetrical density were identified on the mammographic films.

1.4. A sparsely populated mass with no specific character in a low-density area

Given the paucity of signs of infiltration specific to CLI, any ectopic or atypical "glandular" location (internal quadrants, axillary extension, etc.) should attract attention and prompt the patient to undergo additional imaging. The latter easily removes any doubt by showing a constant suspicious mass under localized compression.

1.5. Multifocalite

One of the distinctive features of CLI is the multifocal involvement of the breast parenchyma.

Histology reveals multiple cellular aggregates within the peri-lobular connective stroma.
In a series of 130 CLI cases, Tot et al [27] found 49% uni-focal involvement, 12% multifocal involvement and 28% diffuse infiltration, the latter form having a very poor prognosis.
In our series, multifocal involvement was noted in 2 patients (6.9%).

1.6. Micro-calcification

Microcalcifications, which are easily detected on mammography, are rarely seen in CLI. They are usually round, punctiform or even powdery and polymorphous. The frequency of microcalcifications associated with CLI varies from 1 to 25% [41].
The absence of microcalcifications in CLI is an additional factor contributing to the low sensitivity of mammography in detecting these tumour types. Microcalcifications may also reflect an associated ductal component.
In our series, microcalcifications were detected in 8 cases (26.66%).

1.7. Skin changes

These were reported in certain series: skin thickening, progressive reduction in breast size. This appearance would be correlated with a large mass with a poor prognosis.
In our series, skin signs such as skin retraction, skin thickening and nipple retraction were observed respectively in one patient (3.33%), 4 patients (13.33%) and two patients (6.66%).

1.8. Occult mammograms

The results are highly variable: up to 50% of cases in some series [45]. Occult mammography is defined as the absence of any individualisable abnormality on the 4 basic screening images. Most often, these are dense breasts (BIRADS densities c and d). In this case, ultrasound reveals lesions in 80 to 90% of cases [42].
Apart from dense breasts, CLI may cause opacity of the same density as the surrounding glandular tissue (even in a low-density breast) and without signs of infiltration. In this case, breast ultrasound, thanks to its high sensitivity, can help to correct the diagnosis by showing a tumour mass or a suspicious image.
In short, the mammographic appearance of CLI is often subtle. Despite the apparently low sensitivity of mammography in detecting CLI, the way in which these tumours manifest themselves on mammographic films is well documented.

1.9. Tomosynthesis

The arrival of tomosynthesis represents a technological turning point involving an innovative image acquisition process (information processing, modification of dosimetry and its calculation, use of powerful reconstruction algorithms)

[43].

Tomosynthesis provides a volumetric approach to the breast, and its main contribution is to avoid normal fibroglandular superimpositions, which is particularly noticeable in the visualisation of lesions in women with high-density breasts, and in the differentiation of superimposed structures.

The addition of tomosynthesis to mammography makes it possible to detect smaller, less invasive lesions that would not have been diagnosed by mammography alone. Several studies have demonstrated the value of tomosynthesis in detecting masses and their contours, architectural distortions and asymmetrical density. Indeed, several authors have demonstrated that tomosynthesis enhances the performance of 2D mammography for the detection and characterisation of CLI [43--46].

The mammographic characteristics of CLI and the limits of each modality are detailed in the table below.

Table III: Mammographic aspects of CLI in different series

	Micro Calcifications	Mass Spiculee	Focal asymmetry of density	Isolated distortion	Negatives	Other Signs
Evans et al [39]	11%	60%	9%	20%	-	-
Hillern [40]	-	53%	4%	16%	16%	7%
Le Gal [47]	-	50%	19%	18%	-	12%
Our study	26.66%	74.35%	-	23.33%	-	26.66%

2. Breast ultrasound

Ultrasound is a useful and essential adjunct to mammography. CLI has no specific ultrasound characteristics that can be used to distinguish it from CCI. The sensitivity of ultrasound in detecting CLI varies between 68% and 98%. The false-negative rate can be as high as 12%. The use of ultrasound as a complement to mammography had considerably increased the detection rate of CLI. Butler et al examined 81 mammographically subtle or invisible lesions and found that 87.7% of these were easily detectable by ultrasound. They also reported ultrasound abnormalities in 73.3% of cases in the presence of clinical abnormalities and normal mammograms [48].

Ultrasound had been shown to provide a more accurate measure of the size of the tumour mass compared with mammography and clinical examination. These findings led to changes in surgical management in 18% of cases in the series reported by Berg and colleagues [49]. Ultrasound is superior to mammography in the detection of multicentricity and multifocality, the sensitivity of which was approximately 21% in the Selinko series [50].

The most commonly described ultrasound features of CLI are a hypoechoic, irregular mass with a long vertical axis. The irregular contours are blurred, angular or microlobulated. The contents are usually heterogeneous. Posterior attenuation is inconstant, but classic. The hyperechogenic halo appears to be a determinant sign and is frequently found in Skaane [33].

Selinko et al [50] described the appearance of 62 cases of CLI. The most common sonographic appearance was a hypoechoic mass associated with posterior shadowing in 36 cases (58%), and without posterior attenuation in 17 cases (27%). A posterior acoustic shadow without mass was described in 07 cases (17%). A relatively well circumscribed mass was described in only one case (2%) and one lesion (2%) was sonographically occult. These findings, although not specific to CLI, were found in our study population.

Butler studied whether ultrasound could be useful specifically in CLI that are occult on mammography: in fact 73% of mammographically invisible CLI tumours were identified by an ultrasound-guided examination. Furthermore, 92% of "mammographically subtle" tumours were validated by ultrasound [51].

These studies reinforce the fact that, in the context of a suspicious physical examination result combined with a 'normal' mammogram, ultrasound is a very valuable addition to the diagnosis of CLI.

Ultrasound can also be used to perform echo-guided biopsies or punctures, increasing diagnostic yield. It also plays an important role in detecting axillary lymph nodes with suspicious morphological characteristics. Boughey et al [52] showed that axillary ultrasound had a sensitivity of 52%, a specificity of 79%, a positive predictive value of 73% and a negative predictive value of 61% in the detection of lymph node metastasis.

In our series, there had been no biopsy of ultrasound-suspicious axillary adenopathy and no correlation with histological data. Breast ultrasound was combined with mammography in all patients. It showed an uncircumscribed hypoechoic image in 84.61% associated with posterior acoustic attenuation images in 51.72% of cases.

3. Magnetic resonance imaging

The low sensitivity of mammography and ultrasound in the radiographic detection and estimation of the tumour size of CLI, due to the insidious infiltration mode of this tumour, has led to interest in other radiological modalities to improve early detection and management to avoid therapeutic failure.

Because of its high sensitivity, estimated at 93% [53,54], which is greater than that of mammography and ultrasound, MRI has established itself as the essential examination for assessing the local extension of CLI [55]. Indeed, several studies have confirmed the high sensitivity of MRI compared with other radiological examinations in the assessment of locoregional tumour extension. However, a number of preliminary studies and general reviews have highlighted the possibility of false-negative MRI in CLI.

In some prospective studies, the sensitivity of MRI can reach 95 and 97% [56]. It is superior to the other diagnostic modalities which represent respectively: 65 to 98% for clinical examination, 81 to 98% for mammography and 68 to 98% for ultrasound [57].

CLI manifests itself on MRI in several ways:

3.1. Mass

The most common morphology on MRI is mass-like enhancement, with an incidence of 21% to 95%. It is most often a single mass, irregular in shape and spiculated in outline [58].

3.2. Non-mass enhancement (RNM) and foci

The second type of image is the non-mass enhancement.

The lesions observed are either multiple foci linked by linear enhancement, which corresponds histologically to a discontinuous tumour with cells in single file, or cluster enhancement, which is correlated with small clusters of cells separated by normal breast tissue.

This type of enhancement was present in two patients in our study.

There are also regional, segmental, ductal and diffuse enhancements which correspond in mammography to images of architectural distortion or asymmetries of density [59; 60].

3.3. Asymmetry and architectural distortion in MRI

In the literature, distortions in MRI are much rarer than in mammography.

Schelfout et al [58] described only three cases of distortion identified by MRI: the first was a palpable mass with no abnormality on conventional assessment, and the other two were a distortion image on mammography with no clinical or ultrasound abnormality.

Phillips et al [61] described a case of asymmetry without contrast.

3.4. Normal MRI

It is rare to find a normal MRI in CLI. According to Schelfout et al [64] only one case of normal MRI was found in their studies, corresponding to mammographic distortion on standard imaging and a circumscribed mass on ultrasound, and this is probably related to the technique and protocol used.

In conclusion, the majority of lesions are seen on MRI as mass-like enhancements with characteristics typical of malignancy (irregular shapes and contours, sometimes spicules).

In cases where the mass is not visible on mammography, the lesion on MRI is shown as non-mass enhancement.

MRI of the breast is strongly recommended by several scientific societies as an essential part of the pre-therapeutic work-up for CLI, as it helps to establish diagnostic certainty, provides a better estimate of the size of lesions, enables multifocality to be detected and the contralateral breast to be explored, all of which contribute to the correct choice of therapeutic strategy.

3.5. Size estimation

According to Parvaiz et al, [62] they did not find a significant difference between the pathological size and the size detected on MRI (p = 0.999).

Boetes et al, showed an underestimation of more than 1 cm in 4 cases and an overestimation of the size in 13% of cases [56].

Parvaiz et al, [62] in their turn found an overestimation of size in 29% of cases but less than 3 mm, which is not significant in clinical practice.

3.6. Detection of additional lesions

According to the meta-analysis by Mann et al [59], additional lesions requiring histological proof were only detected by MRI in 32% of cases in the homolateral breast and in 7% of cases in the contralateral breast.

3.7. Multifocalite estimation

Mann et al [59] carried out a meta-analysis comparing the different imaging modalities in the detection of multifocal lesions; 7% of lesions were overestimated by MRI compared with 3% which were underestimated. In the same study, mammography overestimated multifocality in 3% of cases, underestimated it in 40% and did not identify any lesions in 6%.

3.8. Limitations of MRI

The advantage of MRI is that it can detect additional homolateral and contralateral lesions not detectable by echomammography, enabling the most appropriate therapeutic modality to be chosen.

However, MRI is not without its limitations. Like all radiological examinations, it lacks specificity, which is why biopsy remains essential for any additional lesion detected by MRI.

4. Breast biopsy

Percutaneous biopsies are essential to identify the histological type of tumour.

These techniques have a very low false-negative rate and, particularly in the case of foci of micro-calcifications, make it possible to avoid unnecessary interventions and to be able to propose the "right therapeutic choice" at the outset [63].

5. Anatomopathological study of invasive lobular carcinoma

Anatomopathological examination of the surgical specimens enables a definite diagnosis of the histological type of breast cancer to be made, and the final TNM classification to be established in order to guide therapeutic management and predict the prognosis of the disease.

5.1. Invasive lobular carcinoma

5.1.1. Macroscopy

It usually appears as a whitish or beige lesion with poor boundaries and a firm consistency. Occasionally presents as an induced fat, with fibrous tracts separated by fatty lobules of firm consistency [64].

5.1.2. Microscopy

The classic form of CLI is usually distinguished from its 7 variants: trabecular, tubular, solid, alveolar, kitten-ring, histiocytoid and pleomorphic.

All have in common a cytological appearance corresponding to isolated round cells or cells arranged in single file, more rarely in patches. The cells are monomorphic with round nuclei. The cytoplasm is acidophilic and not very abundant and is often hollow with a secretory vacuole ejecting the nucleus to the periphery [65].

5.2. Classic invasive lobular carcinoma

In its classic form, CLI is characterised by small, round, uniform infiltrating cells, either isolated or arranged in rows. The stroma is abundant and densely fibrous, with perichondrial and perivenous elastosis. A lymphocytic infiltrate is sometimes present, which may hide the neoplastic component.

5.3. Variants of invasive lobular carcinoma

5.3.1. Architectural variants of the CLI

Massive (solid) type: consisting of massive cellular patches with a pseudolymphomatous appearance.

Alveolar type: in the form of small round islands reminiscent of CLIS.

Trabecular type: the veins are thicker than in the classic form, with two or three layers of cells. This variant is rarely isolated.

Fisher tubulolobular type: comprising micro-tubes with a narrow lumen. [65]

5.3.2. CLI cell variants

Histiocytoid cells: these are tumour cells with abundant granular and foamy cytoplasm. They may simulate a granular cell tumour. Considered as a variant of CLI with apocrine differentiation.

Kitten-ring cells: a variety of lobular carcinoma with a significant number of cells accumulating intracytoplasmic mucin. It should be distinguished from colloid carcinoma, although the 2 types sometimes coexist.

Pleomorphic CLI: An aggressive form in menopausal women. The usual architecture of lobular carcinoma is observed. However, the cytonuclear atypia are much more marked, with irregularly sized, highly nucleated nuclei, reduced cytoplasm and increased mitotic activity. E-cadherin is often negative. [66]

6. Assessment of extension

CLI's originality lies in its metastatic mode of dissemination.

According to Chann et al: CLI can spread to unusual sites: peritoma, retroperitoma and hollow viscera. Overall, CLI is characterised by diffuse infiltration of these organs, similar to lymphomas. These particular localisations are seen late in the course of the disease and may go clinically unnoticed [67].

6.1. Clinical examination

The clinical examination is vital for assessing the extent of the disease locally and generally.

The aim of the locoregional examination is to look for :

Fixation of the tumour to the deep plane (pectoral).

Fixation to the superficial plane (cutaneous).

A lesion of the contralateral breast.

Axillary ADPs and their characteristics.

The presence of inflammatory signs.

6.2. . Imaging

According to the recommendations, a work-up for CLI should include [68]:

A chest X-ray.

Hepatic ultrasound.

A bone scan (for tumours larger than 1 cm).

A cerebral or whole-body CT scan may be performed, depending on the presenting signs.

The aim of this assessment is to detect any metastases likely to modify the therapeutic approach.

6.3. Tumour markers

The sensitivity of CA 15.3 varies depending on the metastatic site.

It is more important for hepatic localisations and pleural effusions, and secondarily for bone and lung metastases. The sensitivity of CA 15.3 is poor for cerebral metastases [69].

Metastatic forms of emboli are generally rare in CLI. According to Fondriner et al [70], metastatic forms of emboli have been found in 0.5% of cases.

In our series, only one patient consulted at the metastatic stage (hepatic location), which represented 3.33%.

7. Treatment

The therapeutic options for CLI of the breast vary according to the size, stage, presence or absence of metastases and histoprognostic factors of the tumour.

Breast cancer treatment is based on two components:

Locoregional treatment: Resection of the primary tumour and draining lymph nodes.

General treatment: to treat any distant sub-clinical spread.

7.1 Therapeutic methods

7.1.1. Surgery

Surgery consists of removal of the tumour (conservative treatment) or removal of the whole breast (radical treatment) followed by axillary lymph node dissection.

7.1.1.1. Tumour surgery

a. Conservative surgery

Over the last 40 years, the surgical management of breast cancer has undergone enormous changes, and breast conservation has become the most widely adopted strategy for the majority of patients because prospective randomised trials have shown survival rates equivalent to ICC [71].

The examination must be wide, covering the entire glandular thickness, right down to the plane of the pectoralis major, with clean, straight sections.

In general, skin resection of the tumour is not necessary, unless there is a suspicion of invasion.

The margin of the exeresis is a factor in determining the risk of local recurrence. In practice, it should be all the more important when the patient is young, the tumour is aggressive (grade, mitotic index, emboli) and there are associated lesions such as CIS [72].

During this time, several studies have concluded that it is often necessary to modify the initial therapeutic indication in CLI.

According to the series by Yeatman et al [73], the indication for conservative treatment should be changed to mastectomy twice as frequently as for invasive ductal cancers because of the anatomopathological data and underestimation of the initial size of the tumour.

In a retrospective study of 131 patients, Hussien et al [74] compared the rate of local recurrence after conservative treatment versus mastectomy: after 8 years, they observed that local recurrence in the case of conservative treatment was much more frequent than in the case of mastectomy: 42% versus 5%.

b. Radical surgery

The Patey procedure involves removal of the entire gland (including the nipple plate) followed by lymph node dissection.

The overriding imperative of mastectomy is the completeness of glandular exeresis. The cutaneous-glandular detachment must be sufficiently superficial to remove any glandular hotspots, but it must imperatively respect the subdermal vascular network to avoid skin necrosis.

7.1.1.2. Lymph node removal

a. Axillary dissection

It is an important element of locoregional control and is used to staging breast cancer. It has both prognostic and therapeutic value.
Monobloc axillary dissection is the standard technique, but in the case of conservative treatment, it is often separated from the initial incision.
A successful cure is said to have included 10 or more lymph nodes, otherwise repeat surgery is deemed necessary.
The axillary curage should be limited by the lower edge of the axillary vein at the top, the latissimus dorsi muscle to the outside and in depth, and the latissimus dorsi muscle to the inside, respecting the pedicle of the latissimus dorsi (lower scapular) and the nerve of the latissimus dorsi.
Axillary curage may be complicated at a later stage, resulting in lymphaemia, pain or stiffness of the shoulder. [75]

b. The axillary sentinel lymph node

This technique is used to replace curage only for small cancers.
This involves searching for the first lymph node relay (1 to 2 lymph nodes), by injecting a lymphophilic product peri-areolar, which will drain down to the first lymph node, enabling it to be located.
If the sentinel lymph node is invaded, conventional lymph node dissection is carried out; if not, dissection and its sequelae can be avoided, and the morbidity and length of hospital stay can be reduced.

7.1.1.3. Breast reconstruction

It can be carried out in 2 ways: immediate breast reconstruction (IBR) or secondary breast reconstruction (SBR).
The RMI is carried out at the same time as the mastectomy.
However, the RMS is carried out 6 to 12 months after the end of complementary treatments (radiotherapy or chemotherapy) and in particular parietal radiotherapy [76].
There are currently 6 valid surgical techniques for breast reconstruction:

- breast prosthesis alone.
- breast prosthesis after skin expansion.
- dorsalis major muscle flap with prosthesis.
- autologous" dorsalis major muscle flap without prosthesis.
- rectus abdominis muscle flap (TRAM).
- micro anastomosis abdominal fat flap (DIEP).

These techniques differ from one another in terms of the complexity of the operation, the risks of complications and failure (which are greater in the case of smokers) and the quality of the aesthetic result.

7.1.2. Chemotherapy

7.1.2.1. Adjuvant chemotherapy

The aim of adjuvant chemotherapy is to eradicate micrometastases in selected patients at risk, in order to prevent relapse and improve prognosis.

Some authors indicate that patients with CLI are not preferred candidates for chemotherapy, mainly due to their advanced age, greater oestrogen receptor positivity and less lymph node involvement compared with CIN [77,78].

In our series, adjuvant chemotherapy was carried out in 76.66% of patients.

a. Duration of treatment

Currently, the European Society for Medical Oncology (ESMO) recommends at least 4 cycles, i.e. a duration of adjuvant chemotherapy of 18 to 24 weeks [79].

7.1.2.2. Neoadjuvant chemotherapy

Neoadjuvant chemotherapy consists of administering a cytotoxic treatment based on anthracyclines and taxanes prior to surgery.

A number of studies have shown that CLI is not sensitive to neoadjuvant chemotherapy.

According to Jamie Wagner [80], CLI patients undergoing conservative surgery after neoadjuvant chemotherapy tend to have unhealthy margins requiring a second operation.

In our series, neoadjuvant chemotherapy was used in 13.33% of cases.

7.1.3. Radiotherapy

Radiotherapy can be given as a curative treatment in addition to radical or conservative surgery, or as a palliative treatment at various metastatic sites.

7.1.3.1. Post-operative radiotherapy

It significantly reduces the risk of local recurrence at 5 years: according to the study by Diepenmaat et al [81], recurrence was only 2.1% for patients who received radiotherapy after mastectomy despite their advanced stage, compared with 8.5% for patients who did not receive radiotherapy.

This study confirms that treatment with mastectomy and radiotherapy is a highly effective combination for reducing the risk of local recurrence in CLI.

These results confirm the radiosensitive nature of CLI, and could lead to the conclusion that any patient with CLI should benefit from post-operative radiotherapy, whatever the stage of the tumour.

In the case of distant metastases, the use of locoregional treatment either by surgery, radiotherapy, or a combination of the two, to avoid complications of metastases and prevent secondary dissemination is still under discussion.

However, this option could be particularly interesting in the case of CLI, since overall survival after the diagnosis of metastases is significantly longer than with CINS.

In our series, 93.33% of patients received post-surgery radiotherapy.

7.1.4. Hormonotherapy

This is an important step in treatment, as CLI is a hormone-sensitive tumour.

7.1.4.1. Goal

There are three objectives:

Acting on micro-metastasis to improve overall survival.

Improve locoregional control by facilitating surgery and/or radiotherapy.

Preventing breast cancer.

7.1.4.2. Methods of administration

Hormone therapy is indicated for hormone-sensitive tumours (HR+: for estrogen receptors, ER+ and/or progesterone receptors, PR+).

In the literature, more than 90% of CLI are hormone receptor positive, whereas only 5-14% of CLI are clinically HER-2 positive [82].

Pestalozzi et al [32] analysed the results of 15 groups of international breast cancer studies, comprising 667 CLI and 8607 CCI, and found that only half the patients in each group received hormonal therapy, despite the fact that the majority of CLI were hormone receptor positive (76.4% vs. 59.5% of CLI and CCI, respectively).

The risk of recurrence was significantly lower in patients with CLI, but after 6 years of treatment, the risk of recurrence increases considerably, reaching 54% compared with other histological types of breast cancer.

Rakha et al [83] found similar results to those presented by Pestalozzi et al. Patients with CLI had fewer recurrences than patients with CINS in the 10 years following the start of hormone therapy, but revolution was not sufficiently favourable after 10 years.

On the basis of the data from these studies, we can see that the prognosis for CLI is not always better than for CINS in the long term, even after hormone therapy.

In our series, 93.33% had received hormone therapy.

7.1.5. Targeted therapy

Advances in molecular biology and oncogenesis are contributing to the development of targeted cancer therapies.

This technique uses anti antigen antibodies located on the surface of cancer cells, and molecules capable of blocking enzymatic reactions essential to the division of the cancer cell.

A number of studies have focused on the contribution of these therapies to the adjuvant and neoadjuvant treatment of CLI.

Targeted therapy studies in CLI have focused on FGFR1 as a major therapeutic target.

The REIS-FILHO study [84] identified an amplification of FGFR1 during CLI, suggesting the study of new molecules or antibodies directed against FGFR1.
In our series, 13.33% had benefited from the targeted therapy.

8. Prognostic factors

8.1. Clinical factors

8.1.1. Age

Age is one of the predictors of breast cancer.
CLI mainly affects older women, with a poor prognosis and low life expectancy even in young women aged 35, as the tumour is more aggressive at this age and invades fairly quickly.
CLI is most often classified as high-grade at the time of diagnosis.

8.1.2. Evolutionary stage

CLIs are generally large at diagnosis and often develop quiescently.
Approximately 18% of invasive lobular tumours are classified as stage II (T2N0) at diagnosis, compared with 13% of ductal tumours, leading to the conclusion that lobular carcinomas are less aggressive [85].
Size is the major factor in the transition from stage I to II, and not because of lymph node metastases, given the low lymphatic dissemination in CLI.
MORENO-ELOLA et al [86] found that CINS had a higher potential for axillary lymph node metastasis than CLI (37% versus 32% respectively) despite a larger tumour size in CLI, demonstrating that there is no correlation between tumour size (T) and lymph node invasion (N).
In conclusion, in CLI, axillary lymph node invasion should be considered as a prognostic factor rather than tumour size.

8.2. Histological factors

8.2.1. Histological subtype

Histological subtypes are a predictive factor in the prognosis of CLI.
Orvieto E et al [87] studied the prognosis of the different histological subtypes in a series of 530 patients with CLI.
They found that histological variants of CLI had a poorer prognosis and an increased number of distant metastases, compared with the classic form.
In conclusion, histopathological subtyping of CLI is essential as a prognostic element and will therefore condition therapeutic management.

8.2.2. Histopronostic grade

Histopronostic grading depends essentially on the morphology of the tumour cells and the number of mitoses.
Whatever grading system is used, all studies conclude that the higher the grade, the worse the prognosis [88].
Histopronostic grade is therefore a major prognostic factor in breast cancer, and

has a significant impact on overall survival and management.

High grade SBR III in the Scarf-Bloom and Richardson (SBR) score represents a poor prognostic factor and is associated with a high risk of metastatic spread, particularly to the liver and lungs.

The majority of CLIs are classified as grade 2, due to moderate nuclear pleomorphism and low mitotic activity.

In our series, the rate of SBR II grade tumours is 73.33%, followed by SBR I 23.33%.

8.2.3. Histological lymph node involvement

Numerous studies have concluded that node-negative patients have a better prognosis than those with locoregional metastases.

Mac Grogan et al [89] have reported that the characteristics of the cells in CLI (uniform appearance of the cells, absence of cellular atypia and low mitotic rate) make the detection of tumour cells in the lymph nodes difficult, leading to an underestimation of lymph node dissemination for this type of cancer, which justifies more frequent use of immunohistochemistry in cases of doubt.

Fortunato et al [14] found that the rate of lymph node involvement in CLI was 33%.

In our series, the rate of axillary invasion was 72.4%.

8.2.4. Vascular emboli

Vascular emboli represent a poor prognostic factor. Many believe that the presence of vascular emboli is less frequent in CLI, which may be a good prognostic factor for this type of cancer.

In our study, there were no cases of vascular emboli.

8.2.5. Immunohistochemistry

Immunohistochemical studies can be used to identify tumours with an aggressive tendency, enabling the most appropriate therapeutic strategy to be adopted.

8.2.5.1. Hormone receptors (Table IV)

These are intracellular receptors that bind restrogen and progesterone. Their presence gives the tumour a hormone-sensitive character.

The vast majority of CLI express restrogen and progesterone receptors, making them sensitive to hormonal treatment and improving their prognosis [90].

The table below compares the hormone receptor levels found in our series with the literature.

Table IV: Hormone receptor levels in patients with CLI.

Authors	Number of patients	BR Positive(%)	Positive PR(%)
Korhonen et al [34]	295	92%	72%
Coradini et al [91]	67	96%	76%

Our study	30	93.33%	86.6%

8.2.5.2. The C-erbB-2 (or HER-2) oncogene

A proto-oncogene located on the long arm of chromosome 17q21, it is often overexpressed in 30% of breast cancers and has been shown to be a poor prognostic factor.

It is involved in breast cancerogenesis through amplification and/or overexpression of its product, the HER-2 protein, which is used as a monitoring tool for metastatic breast cancers expressing HER-2 [92].

Overexpression of the HER-2 protein to identify patients who will benefit from the therapy targeted by Trastuzumab (Herceptin®).

In our study, overexpression of the HER2 protein was noted in 4 cases.

8.2.5.3. KI 67

The KI-67 antigen is one of the proliferation markers.

The mean positive value of Ki67 cells in breast tumours is 15%.

A strong correlation between Ki67 expression and survival has also been reported.

For infiltrating lobular carcinomas, the proliferation index is generally low, which is associated with a better prognosis. [93]

In our series, only 3 patients had positive KI67 values.

9. Prognosis

9.1. Survival

Once properly treated, CLI usually progresses favourably.

MORENO-ELOLA et al [86] carried out a multidisciplinary descriptive study, retrospective and prospective, in various centres, on a population of 404 patients with invasive carcinoma of the breast of pure or mixed lobular type. In this study, overall survival was 89.4% at 1 year, 86.1% at 2 years, 81.8% at 4 years, 77.2% at 6 years and finally 65.5% at 8 years. Overall survival at 10 years was 65%, and 50% at 17 years.

In our study, overall 5-year survival was estimated at 77.3%.

9.2. Metastases

CLI metastasises via the hematogenic or lymphatic route. Its mode of metastatic spread is different from that of CINS.

CLI frequently metastasises to the peritoneum, retroperitoneum, bone, meninges, stomach, digestive tract, bone marrow and gynaecological organs, with fewer pleuropulmonary metastases [94].

Fondriner et al [70] compared the metastatic revolution of ductal and lobular carcinomas of the breast from two matched series (376 patients), and found that hepatic, pulmonary and cerebral metastases were more frequent in NICC, whereas digestive, peritoneal and gynaecological metastases were much more characteristic of CLI. There was no difference in overall or event-free survival between the two populations. These results therefore confirm the differences in metastatic evolution and raise the question of the unsuitability of the extension tests currently proposed for CLI.

Knowledge of the metastatic spread of CLI is essential for the interpretation of images during extension work-up, in order to detect a metastatic location of the disease.

In our series, only one patient had a secondary hepatic location at the time of diagnosis.

10. Monitoring

The aim of monitoring is to detect any local or distant recurrence of the tumour as early as possible, and also to detect and treat any side-effects of the treatment.

10.1. Local and regional surveillance

The most useful form of screening, it is based essentially on clinical examination and mammography.

A clinical examination is carried out every 3 months during the first year and every 6 months thereafter for 5 years, then once a year for life. This examination covers both breasts, the chest wall and satellite lymph nodes.

The practice of self-examination, which requires prior education of the patient.

The 1st mammogram should be carried out 6 months after the end of treatment, and then repeated every year. It should also involve the contralateral breast, given the frequency of contralateral cancers in CLI.

10.2. General surveillance

The aim is to look for any distant metastases; more than half of metastases are discovered by clinical examination and questioning, and a chest X-ray and tumour marker assay should be carried out every year. A gynaecological examination is also essential every year, especially in women on Tamoxifen, with pelvic ultrasound performed whenever there are clinical symptoms.

Other paraclinical examinations to be carried out in the event of warning signs are :

- a bone scan.
- hepatic ultrasound, hepatic assessment
- a cerebral CT scan.

Tumour markers can be used to detect sub-clinical metastases, but they do not have a clear impact on overall survival.

11. Summary and limitations of the study

CLI is a particular and rare variety of breast cancer whose incidence has increased markedly in recent years. We found the clinical and radiological features to be varied and largely consistent with the literature. Nevertheless, this work would be meaningless if it did not make it possible to draw up certain proposals which will contribute to the improvement of current practice by highlighting solutions to the problems posed in the results and discussion section. These recommendations are aimed at improving the management of CLI in terms of assessment and treatment prospects.

Given the ways in which CLI is disseminated, it would seem useful to adapt the extension work-up in view of the metastatic spread of CLI, which differs from that of CIN, with more frequent involvement of the digestive tract, stomach, ovaries and meninges, which may pose a problem in terms of monitoring, We note that only one patient in our series benefited from exploration by thoraco-abdominopelvic CT scan, none of the patients was explored by endovaginal pelvic ultrasound to look for ovarian metastases, and breast MRI was performed in only 3 patients.

We also stressed the importance of MRI, which is playing an increasingly important role in the management of CLI, because of its proven superiority over mammography and ultrasound in terms of detecting multifocalities and multicentricities, and providing a more accurate assessment of the extent of the disease, enabling the right therapeutic choice to be made.

In fact, the progress of new anti-cancer therapeutic technologies such as target therapy, which targets the cancerogenes involved in the genesis of CLI, offers the prospect of a new strategy in the management of this histological type; and intraoperative radiotherapy represents a genuine technological revolution and is a recognised option for the management of breast cancers with a low risk of recurrence. The literature has shown that, at 5 years post-operatively, it makes it possible to obtain a low local recurrence rate, even similar to that of conventional external radiotherapy, without increasing skin toxicity, and makes it possible to improve patients' quality of life.

5 CONCLUSION

Invasive lobular carcinoma (ILC) of the breast is a rare histological entity, accounting for between 5 and 15% of all breast cancers. It is the second most common histological type, after non-specific infiltrating carcinoma (NISC), and its incidence has risen sharply in recent years.

The aims of our work were to describe the anatomical and clinical features of CLI, as well as the treatment methods, to clarify the role of breast imaging in positive diagnosis, and to identify the main prognostic factors for CLI of the breast.

We conducted a retrospective descriptive study of 30 observations of CLI of the breast collected in the Obstetric Gynecology Department of the Monastir Maternity and Neonatology Centre over a 10-year period from 01 January 2008 to 31 December 2017.

The incidence of CLI in our study was 4%, rising from 2% in 2008 to 7% in 2017. The mean age at onset of CLI was 53.43 years. Oral contraceptives were taken in 33.33% of cases and 53.33% of patients were menopausal.

A breast nodule was the most frequent warning sign and was observed in 25 cases (83.33%) with an average size of 3.31 cm.

Mammography showed a bifocal mass in 5 patients (17.24%), a unifocal mass in 21 patients (72.41%) and a bilateral mass in 3 patients (10.35%), 2 of whom had multifocal lesions. The mass had spiculated contours in 29 cases (74.35%) and an area of architectural disorganisation was observed in 7 patients (23.33%). Microcalcifications were observed in 8 patients (26.66%).

Ultrasound showed a hypoechogenic image that was not circumscribed in 84.61% of cases, associated with posterior acoustic attenuation images in 51.72% of cases. Radiological assessment classified the lesions as ACR5 in 63.33% and ACR 4 in 36.66%.

MRI is superior to other radiological examinations in assessing the locoregional extent of the tumour. It provides a better estimate of lesion size, screening for multifocal disease and exploration of the contralateral breast, and helps to guide the choice of treatment. In our series, MRI was indicated in 3 patients and showed non-mass enhancement in two cases.

The majority of tumours were classified as T2 in 44.44% of cases, T1 in 38.88%, T4 in 11.11% and T3 in 5.57%. N0 in 63.33% of cases and N1 in 36.66%. M1 in 3.33% and M0 in 96.66%.

Anatomopathological study of the surgical specimen showed unifocal CLI in 54.84%, bifocal CLI in 19.36% and multifocal CLI in 25.8% of cases. Lymph node involvement was confirmed in 72.41% of cases. The majority of tumours were classified as SBR2 (74.2% of cases), SBRI in 22.58% of cases and SBRIII in only one case (3.22%). Estrogenic and progestogenic hormone receptors were positive in 93.55% and 87.1% of cases respectively. Overexpression of the HER2 gene was identified in 4 tumours (12.9%). KI67 was found to be greater than 20% in 3 patients.

Patey-type radical surgery was performed initially in 61.33% of cases, while 19.35% of tumours underwent conservative treatment and 19.35% underwent salvage mastectomy. Neoadjuvant chemotherapy was given in 4 patients (13.33%) and adjuvant chemotherapy in 23 cases (76.66%). Twenty-eight patients (93.33%) had received adjuvant radiotherapy and hormonal therapy.

In our series, the overall 5-year survival rate was estimated at 77.3%.

CLI poses a definite diagnostic problem and its incidence is rising sharply, which could be explained by the increase in the prescription of hormone replacement therapy and oral contraception. In the majority of series, patients with CLI are older than those with CINS.

The nodule is the most frequent warning sign, as demonstrated in several series.

CLI is characterised by multifocal and bilateral lesions, which are more common than CINS.

On mammography, CLI is most often seen as a spiculated mass or a patch of architectural distortion, while microcalcifications are not common.

The ultrasound images most commonly described in the literature in CLI are mainly an irregular hypoechogenic mass with large vertical axes. Posterior attenuation is inconstant but classic.

Despite its cost and limited availability, MRI is playing an increasingly important role in the management of CLI, due to its proven superiority over mammography and ultrasound in terms of detecting multifocalities and multicentricities, and providing a more accurate assessment of the extent of the disease, enabling the therapeutic choice to be made.

Therapeutically, there are few particularities compared with NSCLC. However, neoadjuvant chemotherapy is probably less recommended if the tumour is operable, and hormonal therapy appears to be an essential treatment in the therapeutic armoury.

CLI is characterised by a metastatic spread that differs from that of CINS, with more frequent involvement of the digestive tract, stomach, ovaries and meninges, which may pose a problem for its surveillance and mean that its extension work-up needs to be adapted.

CLI appears to have a good prognosis, as it is often of low histopronostic grade, and its course is often insidious, with hormone receptors being positive in the majority of cases. Nevertheless, its prognosis does not appear to differ from that of CIN in the long term.

In conclusion, CLI represents a particular variety of breast carcinoma, and this study attempted to describe its various epidemiological, clinical, radiological and therapeutic characteristics, which were largely consistent with the literature. In addition, advances in new anti-cancer therapeutic technologies, such as target therapies targeting the cancerogenes involved in the genesis of CLI, offer the prospect of a new strategy for managing this histological type and improving its prognosis.

6 REFERENCES

[1] Lee JH, Park S, Park HS, Park BW. Clinicopathological features of infiltrating lobular carcinoma comparing with infiltrating ductal carcinoma: a case control study. World J Surg Oncol. 2010; 8:34.

[2] Orvieto E, Maiorano E, Bottiglieri L, Maisonneuve P, Rotmensz N, Galimberti V, et al. Clinocopathologic characteristics of invasive lobular carcinoma of the breast: results of an analysis of 530 cases from a single institution. Cancer.2008; 113:151:1-20.

[3] Li CI, Anderson BO, Daling JR, Moe RE.Trends in incidence rates of invasive lobular and ductal breast carcinoma. JAMA.2003; 289(11):1421-4.

[4] Ravdin, Peter M. Hormone Replacement Therapy and the Increase in the Incidence of Invasive Lobular Cancer. Breast disease. 2008; 30:3-8

[5] Li CI, Malone KE, Porter PL, Weiss NS, Tang M-TC, Daling JR. Reproductive and anthropometric factors in relation to the risk of lobular and ductal breast carcinoma among women 65-79 years of age. Int J Cancer .2003; 107:647-51.

[6] Chikman B, Lavy R, Davidson T, Wassermann I, Sandban Kj, Siegelmann-Danieli N et al. Factors affecting rise in the incidence of infiltrating lobular carcinoma of the breast. Isr Med Assoc J. 2010; 12(11): 697-700.

[7] . Verkooijen HM1, Fioretta G, Vlastos G, Morabia A, Schubert H, Sappino AP, et al.Important increase of invasivelobular breast cancer incidence in Geneva, Switzerland.Int J Cancer .2003;107: 778-81

[8] Lopez JK, Bassett LW. Invasive lobular carcinoma of the breast: spectrum of mammographic, US, and MR imaging findings. Radiographics. 2009; 29:165-76.

[9] Wasif N, Maggard MA, Ko CY, Giuliano AE. Invasive lobular vs ductal breast cancer: a stage-matched comparison of outcomes. Ann surg oncol.2010; 17:7:1862-19.

[10] Jung, So-Youn, Jeong, Junsoo, Shin, Seung-Ho, ET al.The invasive lobular carcinoma as a prototype luminal a breast cancer: A retrospective cohortstudy. BMC cancer. 2010; 10: 1:664.

[11] Sastre-Garau X, Jouve M, Asselain B. Infiltrating lobular carcinoma of the breast:Clinicopathologic analysis of 975 cases with reference to data onconservative therapy and metastatic patterns.Cancer. 1996; 77:113-20.

[12] Khlifi A, Ziadi S, Trimeche M, Hidar S, Mokni M, Abbassi B et al. Clinicopathological study of lobular carcinomas of the breast in central Tunisia: 74 cases. J afr cancer. 2011.3: 3:155-62.

[13] Li CI, Uribe DJ, Daling JR. Clinical characteristics of different histologic types of breast cancer. Br J Cancer. 2005; 93(9):1046-52.

[14] Fortunato, Lucio, Mascaro, Alessandra, Poccia, Igor et al. Lobular breast cancer: same survival and local control compared with ductal cancer, but should both be treated the same way? Analysis of an institutional data base over a 10year period.Ann surg oncol. 2012; 19: 4:1107-14.

[15] Collaborative Group on Hormonal Factors in Breast Cancer.Menarche, menopause, and breast cancer risk: individual participant meta-analysis, including 118,964 women with breast cancer from 117 epidemiological studies. Lancet Oncol.2012;13:1141-51.

[16] Newcomb PA, Trentham-Dietz A, Hampton JM, Egan KM, Titus,Ernstoff L, Warren Andersen S, Greenberg ER, Willett WC. Late age at first full term birth is strongly associated with lobular breast cancer.Cancer. 2011; 117(9):1946-56.

[17] Li Ci, Malone KE, Porter PL, Weiss NS, Tang MT, Daling JA. Reproductive and anthropometric factors in relation to the risk of lobular and ductal breast carcinoma among women 65-79 years of age. Int.J.Cancer.2003; 107:647-51.

[18] Reeves GK, Beral V, Green J, Gathani T, Bull D. Million Women Study Collaborators: Hormonal therapy for menopause and breast-cancer risk by histological type: a cohort study and meta-analysis. Lancet Oncol. 2006; 7:910-8.

[19] Newcomer LM, Newcomb PA, Trentham-Dietz A, Longnecker MP, Greenberg ER. Oral contraceptive use and risk of breast cancer by histologic type. Int J Cancer. 2003; 106:961-4.

[20] Dupont WD, Page DL, Parl FF, Vnencak-Jones CL, Plummer WD, RadosMS and al .Long-term risk of breast cancer in women with fibroadenoma. N Engl J Med. 1994; 331: 10-15.

[21] Mavaddat N, Barrowdale D, Andrulis IL, Domchek SM, Eccles D, Nevanlinna H, et al. Pathology of breast and ovarian cancers among BRCA1 and BRCA2 mutation carriers: results from the Consortium of Investigators of Modifiers of BRCA1/2 (CIMBA). Cancer Epidemiol Biomark. 2012; 21:134-47.

[22] Corso G, Intra M, Trentin C, Veronesi P, Galimberti V. CDH germline mutations and hereditary lobular breast cancer. Fam Cancer .2016; 15:215-9.

[23] El Alouani C, Khouchani M, Omrani A, Benhmidoune A, Tahri A. Clinicopathological, therapeutic AND evolutionary characteristics of lobular breast cancer in the Marrakech region.Cancer/Radiotherapie.2010;14 (67): 639.

[24] Gump FE.Lobular carcinoma in situ: pathology and treatment. J Cell Biochem .1993; 17:53-8.

[25] Espie M, Hocini H, Cuvier C. Giacchetti S, Bourstyn E. de Roquancour

A. Invasive lobular breast cancer: diagnostic AND evolutionary features. Gynecol obstet fertilite. 2006; 34 (1): 3-7.

[26] Cao, A.-Yong, Huang, Liang, WU, Jiong. Tumor characteristics and the clinical outcome of invasive lobular carcinoma compared to infiltrating ductal carcinoma in a Chinese population. World J Surg Oncol.2012; 10 (1):152.

[27] Tot T. The diffuse type of invasive carcinoma of the breast: morphology and prognosis. Virchows arch. 2003; 443: 718-24

[28] Horn PL, Thompson WD. Risk of contralateral breast cancer: Associations with histologic, clinical, and therapeutic factors .Cancer .1988; 62:412-24.

[29] Polednak AP. Bilateral synchronous breast cancer: a population-based study of characteristics, method of detection, and survival.Surgery.2003; 133:383-9.

[30] Intra M, Rotmensz N, Viale G, Mariani L, Bonanni B, Mauro G et al.Clinicopathologic characteristics of 143 patients with synchronous bilateral invasive breast carcinomas treated in a single institution .Cancer .2004;101: 90512.

[31] Goldflam K, Hunt KK, Gershenwald JE, Singletary SE, Mirza N, Kuerer HM et al.Contralateral prophylactic mastectomy: Predictors of significant histologic findings.Cancer .2004; 101:1977-1986.

[32] Pestalozzi BC, Zahrieh D, Mallon E, Gusterson BA, Price KN, Gelber et al. Distinct clinical and prognostic features of infiltrating lobular carcinoma of the breast: combined results of 15 International Breast Cancer Study Group clinical trials.J Clin Oncol.2008; 26:3006-14.

[33] Skaane P, Skjorten F. Ultrasonographic evaluation of invasive lobular carcinoma. Acta Radiol. 1999; 40:369-75

[34] Korhonen T, Huhtala H Holli K. A comparison of the biological and clinical features of invasive lobular and ductal carcinomas of the breast. Breast Cancer Res Treatment.2004; 85: 23-9.

[35] Porter AJ, Evans EB, Foxcroft LM, Simpson PT, Lakhani SR. Mammographic and ultrasound features of invasive lobular carcinoma of the breast. J Med Imaging Radiat Oncol. 2014; 58:1-10.

[36] Kerlikowske K, Grady D, Barclay J, Sickles EA, Ernster V. Effect of age, breast density, and family history on the sensitivity of first screening mammography. JAMA. 1996; 276:33-8.

[37] Mandelson MT, Oestreicher N, Porter PL, White D, and Finder CA, Taplin SH et al. Breast density as a predictor of mammographic detection: comparison of interval and screen detected cancers. J Natl Cancer Inst. 2000; 92:1081-7.

[38] Berg WA, Gutierrez L, NessAiver MS, Carter WB, Bhargavan M, Lewis RS, et al. Diagnostic accuracy of mammography, clinical examination, US, and MR imaging in preoperative assessment of breast cancer. Radiology. 2004; 233:830-49.

[39] Evans WP, Warren Burhenne LJ, Laurie L, O'Shaughnessy KF, Castellino RA,

Susan G et al. Invasive lobular carcinoma of the breast: mammographic characteristics and computer-aided detection. Radiology. 2002; 225:182-9.

[40] Hilleren DJ, Andersson IT, Lindholm K, Linnell FS. Invasive lobular carcinoma: mammographic findings in a 10-year experience. Radiology.1991; 178:149-54.

[41] Mendelson EB, Harris KM, Doshi N, Tobon H. Infiltrating lobular carcinoma: mammographic patterns with pathologic correlation. Am J Roentgenol.1989;153(2):265-71.

[42] Weinstein S, Greenstein Orel S, Rose Heller, Reynolds C, Brian Czerniecki, LawrenceJ et al. MR imaging of the breast in patients with invasive lobular carcinoma. AJR. 2001; 176:339-406.

[43] Chamming's F, Bouaboul M, Depetiteville MP, Catena V, Rousseau C, Boisserie-Lacroix M. Invasive lobular cancers: conventional imaging and interventional gestures. Imag Femme. 2017; 339-48.

[44] Friedewald SM, Rafferty EA, Rose SL, Durand MA, PlechaDM, Greenberg JS, et al. Breast cancer screening using tomosynthesis in combination with digital mammography. JAMA. 2014;311:2499-507.

[45] Mariscotti G, Durando M, Houssami N, Zuiani C, Martincich L, Londero V, et al. Digital breast tomosynthesis as an adjunctto digital mammography for detecting and characterising invasive lobular cancers: a multi-reader study. Clin Radiol. 2016;71:889-95.

[46] Chamming's F, Kao E, Aldis A, Ferre R, Omeroglu A, ReinholdC, et al. Imaging features and conspicuity of invasive lobular carcinomas on digital breast tomosynthesis. Br J Radiol. 2017;90:190-6.

[47] Le Gal M, Ollivier L, Asselain B, Meunier M, Laurent M, Vielh P, et al. Mammographic features of 455 invasive lobular carcino- mas. Radiology. 1992; 185(3):705-8.

[48] Butler RS, Venta LA, Wiley EL, Ellis RL, Dempsey PJ, Rubin E. Sonographic evaluation of infiltrating lobular carcinoma. Am J Roentgenol.1999; 172:325-30.

[49] Berg W.A, Gutierrez L, NessAiver M.S, Carter W.B, Bhargavan M, Lewis R.S., et al. Diagnostic accuracy of mammography, clinical examination, US, and MR imaging in preoperative assessment of breast cancer. Radiology.

2004; 233: 830-49.

[50] Selinko VL, Middleton LP, Dempsey PJ. Role of sonography in diagnosing and staging invasive lobular carcinoma. J Clin Ultrasound.2004; 32:323-32.

[51] Butler RS, Venta LA, Wiley EL, Ellis RL, Dempsey PJ, Rubin E. Sonographic evaluation of infiltrating lobular carcinoma. Am J Roentgenol.1999; 172:325-30.

[52] Boughey JC, Middleton LP, Harker L. Utility of ultrasound and fine-needle aspiration biopsy of the axilla in the assessment of invasive lobular carcinoma of the breast. Am J Surg.2007; 194:450-5.

[53] C Dratwa, Delphine Sebbag-Sfez, Fabienne Thibault. Breast MRI in infiltrating lobular carcinoma: diagnostic aspects, pretherapeutic workup, evaluation under hormono- or chemo-neoadjuvant.Imag femme.2017; 27 (3):206-215.

[54] Mann RM, Hoogeveen YL, Blickman JG, Boetes C. MRI compared to conventional diagnostic work-up in the detection and evaluation of invasive lobular carcinoma of the breast: a review of existing literature. Breast Cancer Res Treat. 2008; 107:1-14.

[55] Suissa M, Levy L, Tranbaloc P, Chiche JF, Martin B, Skaane P et al. Imaging of invasive lobular cancers. Imag Femme. 2005; 15:129-39.

[56] Boetes C, Veltman J, van Die L, Bult P, Wobbes T, Barentsz JO.The role of MRI in invasive lobular carcinoma. Breast Cancer Res Treat. 2004; 86(1):31-7.

[57] Cawson JN, Law EM, Kavanagh AM. Invasive lobular carcinoma: sonographic features of cancers detected in a breastscreen program. Austral Radiol. 2001; 45(1):25-30.

[58] Schelfout K, Van Goethem M, Kersschot E, Colpaert C, Schelf- hout AM, Leyman P, et al. Contrast-enhanced MR imaging of breast lesions and effect on treatment. Eur J Surg Oncol .2004; 30(5):501-7.

[59] Mann RM, Hoogeveen YL, Blickman JG, Boetes C. MRI compared to conventional diagnostic work-up in the detection and evaluation of invasive lobular carcinoma of the breast: a review of existing literature. Breast Cancer Res Treat. 2008; 107(1):1-14.

[60] Lopez JK, Bassett LW. Invasive lobular carcinoma of the breast: spectrum of mammographic, US, and MR imaging findings. Radiographics. 2009; 29(1):165-76.

[61] Phillips H., Stephen J. Infiltrating lobular carcinoma, part 2: MRI morphology and kinetics. World care clin. 2010; 4(3):1-8.

[62] Parvaiz MA, Yang P, Razia E, Mascarenhas M, Deacon C, Matey P, et al.

Breast MRI in invasive lobular carcinoma: a useful investigation in surgical planning. Breast J .2016; 22(2):143-50.

[63] Seror JY, Antoine M, Scetbon F. Chopier J, Sananes S, Ghenassia C et al. Apport des macrobiopsies stereotaxiques par aspiration dans la stratégie de prise en charge des microcalcifications mammaires: première serie prospective de 115 cas. Gynecologie obstetrique & fertilite. 2000; 28 (11):806-19.

[64] Trojani M, Mac Grogan G.Anatomie pathologique du sein.Encyclopedie medicale ET chirurgicale. [Paris: Elsevier Masson SAS; 1998.

[65] Rakha EA, Ellis IO. Lobular breast carcinoma and its variants.Semin Diagn Pathol.2010; 27:49-61.

[66] Weidner N, Semple JP.Pleomorphic variant of invasive lobular carcinoma of the breast. Hum Pathol .1992; 23(10):1167-71.

[67] CHAN A, PINTILIE M, VALLIS K, GIROURD C, GOSS P. Breast cancer in women <35 years: review of 1002 cases from a single institution. Ann Oncol. 2000; 11(10):1255 -62.

[68] BALU-MAESTRO.C, CHAPELLIER.C, DARCOURT.J, ETTORE.F, RAOUST.I. Imaging in the lymph node AND metastatic extension assessment of breast cancer. J radiol (Paris). 2005; 186:1649-57.

[69] de la Lande B. Current place of CA 15.3 assays in breast cancer. Immuno-anal Biol spec. 2004; 19: 274-278.

[70] Fondriner E, Guerin O, Lorimier G. Etude comparative de l'évolution metastatique des carcinomes canalaires ET lobulaires du sein a partir de deux série appariees (376 patients).Bull cancer. 1997; 84 (12): 1101-7.

[71] Mc Guire KP, Santillan AA, Kaur P. Are mastectomies on the rise? A 13year trend analysis of the selection of mastectomy versus breast conservation therapy in 5865 patients. Ann Surg Oncol. 2009; 16:2682-90.

[72] Houvenaeghel G, Lambaudie E., Buttarelli M. Marge d'exerese dans les cancers infiltrants du sein. Bull Cancer.2008; 95 (12):1161-70.

[73] Yeatman TJ, Cantor AB, Smith TJ, Smith SK, Reintgen DS, Mil- ler MS, et al. Tumor biology of infiltrating lobular carcinoma: Implications for management. Ann Surg. 1995; 222:549-61.

[74] Hussien M, Lioe TF, Finnegan J, Spence RJ. Surgical treat-ment for invasive lobular carcinoma of the breast. Breast. 2003; 12:23-35.

[75] Oliviera JB, Verhaeghea JL, Butarellib M, Marchala F, Houvenaeghel G. Functional anatomy of breast lymphatic drainage: contribution of the sentinel lymph node technique. Ann chir.2006; 131: 608-15.

[76] Horiota J-C, Vrieling C, Brioschi P-A. Reconstructive surgery AND radiotherapy for breast cancer. Imag Femme.2010; 20:18-26.

[77] Frenela J-S, Campone M. Chemotherapy for non-metastatic breast cancer:

state of play in 2010. J Gyncol Obstettr Biol Reprod. 2010; 39: 79-84.
[78] Berry DA, Cirrincione C, Henderson IC, Citron ML, Budman DR, Goldstein LJ et al. Estrogenreceptor status and outcomes of modern chemotherapy for patients with node-positive breast cancer. JAMA .2006; 295:1658-67.
[79] Aebil S, Davidson T, Gruber G, Cardoso F. On behalf of the ESMO Guidelines Working Group Primary breast cancer: ESMO Clinical Practice Guidelines for diagnosis, treatment and follow-up .Clini pract guidelines. Ann Oncol .2011; 22 (sup 6): vi 12-24.
[80] WAGNER J, BOUGHEY JC, GARRETT B. Margin assessment after neoadjuvant chemotherapy in invasive lobular cancer. Am J Surg. 2009; 198(3): 387-91.
[81] DIEPENMAAT LA, SANGEN MJC, POLL-FRANSE LV. The impact of postmastectomy radiotherapy on local control in patients with invasive lobular breast cancer. Radiother Oncol. 2009; 91(1): 49-53.
[82] Yu J, Bhargava R, Dabbs DJ. Invasive lobular carcinoma with extracellular mucin production and HER-2 over expression: a case report and further case studies.Diagn Pathol.2010; 5:36.
[83] Rakha EA, El-Sayed ME, Powe DG, Green AR, Habashy H, Grainge MJ, et al.
Invasive lobular carcinoma of the breast: response to hormonal therapy and outcomes. Eur J Cancer. 2008; 44:73-83.
[84] Reis-Filho JS, Simpson PT, Turner NC, Lambros MB, Jone C, Mackay A et al. FGFR1 emerges as a potential therapeutic target for lobular breast carcinomas.ClinCancer Res. 2006; 12 (22): 6652-62.
[85] yeatman TJ, Cantor AB, Smith TJ. Tumor biology of infiltrating lobular carcinoma. Implications for management. Ann Surg. 1995; 222(4):549-61.
[86] Moreno-Elola A, Roman JM, Aguilar A, Hernandez A, Martin M, Diaz Rubio E et al.Prognostic factors in invasive lobular carcinoma of the breast: a multivariate analysis. A multicentre study after seventeen years of follow-up. Ann Chir Gyn oncol.1999; 88(4):252-8.
[87] Orvieto E, Maiorano E, Bottiglieri L, Maisonneuve P, Rotmensz N, Galimberti V et al. Clinicopathologic characteristics of invasive lobular carcinoma of the breast: results of an analysis of 530 cases from a single institution.Cancer.2008;113(7):1511- 20.
[88] Buchanan CL, Flynn LW, Murray MP, Darvishian F, Cranor ML, Fey JV et al. Is pleomorphic lobular carcinoma really a distinct clinical entity? J Surg Oncol.2008; 98(5):314-7.
[89] MacGrogan G, Jollet I, Huet S, Sierankowski G, Picot V, Bonichon F et

al. Comparison of quantitative and semiquantitative methods of assessing MIB-1 with the S-phase fraction in breast carcinoma.Mod Pathol .1997; 10:769-76.
[90] Azria D, Lemanski C, Zouhair A , Gutowski M , Belkacemi Y , Dubois JB et al.Concomitant adjuvant hormone therapy for breast cancer: state of the art. Cancer/Radiother .2004; 8 (3): 188-96.
[91] Coradini D, Pellizzaro C, Veneroni S, Ventura L, Daidone MG.
Infiltrating ductal and lobular breast carcinomas are characterised by different interrelationships among markers related to angiogenesis and hormone dependence. Br J Cancer .2002; 87:1105-11.
[92] Tapia C, Schraml P, Simon R. HER2 analysis in breastcancer: reduced immunoreactivity in FISH non-informative cancer biopsies.Int j oncol. 2004; 25 (6):1551-7.
[93] Varga Z, Mallon E. Histology and immunophenotype of invasive lobular breast cancer: daily practice and pitfalls. Breast Dis. 2009;30:15-9.
[94] Petrausch U, Pestalozzi B C. Distinct Clinical and Prognostic Features of Invasive Lobular Breast Cancer.Breast dis.2008; 30 (1): 39-44

7 APPENDICES

Appendix 1

ACR Birads classification 5th edition

HI-KAIIS 0	**Need Additional imaging Evaluation and/or Prior Mammograms For (ompartson:**
Further imaging evaluation (eg additional views or ultrasound) or retrieval of prior examinations is required J Aditional imaging audio arc completed. a final a "c>чтпи is marie.	
HI-RAIK 1	**Segative:**
J There o nothing to comment on * The breast v arc symmetric and no masses. architectural distortion or suspicious cakification" arc present	
BI-RADS 2	**Benign Finding:**
J Follow up alter breast conservative surgery J Involuting, calcified fibroadenomas J Multiple large, rod-like calcifications J Intranummary lymph nodes J Vascular calcifications * Implants Architectural distortion clearly related Io prior surgery * Fat-containing lesions such as oil cysts, lipomas, galactoceles and mised-dctisrty hamartomas. They all have charactcnsticallv benign appearances, and muv be labeled with confidence	
BI-RADS Л	**Probably Benign F hiding Initial Short-Inters al Follow-Ip Suggested:**
A finding placed in this category should have Ices than a 2% nsk of malignancy V Nonpalpabic. circumscribed mass on a baseline mammogram **iunless** it can be shown Io be a cyst, an intramammary lymph node, or another benign finding I. J Focal asy nimctry which becomes less dense on spot compression view ✓ Solitary group of punctate cak ilicalums	
BI-RAll's 4	**Suspicious A finer mail tv - Biops s Should Be Considered:**
has a wide range of probability of By subdividing Category 4 into ■ indicated within this category so course of action	malignancy <2 ■ 95%). A. 4B and 4C . it is encouraged that relevant probabilities for malignancy be the patient and her phy sician can make an informed decision on the ultimate
BI-RADS5	**Highly Suggestive of Malignancy. Appropriate Action Should Be Taken:**
BI-RADS 5 must he reserved lor findings that are classic breast cancers, with a >954 likelibixid of malignancy The current rationale for using category S tv that if the percutaneous tissue diagnosis is nonmalignant. this automatically should be considered as discordant J Spiculaled. irregular highdensity mass * Segmental or linear arrangement of fine linear cak'ificallons * Irregular spiculaled mass w ith associated pleomorphic calcifications	

Appendix 2

TNM classification of breast cancer, 7th edition 2010, and UICC stage

The TNM system distinguishes between the pre-therapeutic clinical stage graded "cTNM" and the post-surgical anatomopathological stage graded "pTNM".

PRIMARY TUMOUR T

Tx: the primary tumour cannot be assessed

T0: the primary tumour is not palpable

- Tis: carcinoma in situ
- Tis (DCIS): ductal carcinoma in situ
- Tis (CLIS): lobular carcinoma in situ
- Tis (Paget): Paget's disease of the nipple without underlying tumour
- NB: Paget's disease associated with a tumour is classified according to the size of the tumour.

T1: tumour < 2 cm in its largest dimension

Tlmic: microinvasion < 1 mm in its largest dimension

- T1a: 1 mm < tumour < 5 mm in its largest dimension
- T1b: 5 mm < tumour < 1 cm in its largest dimension
- T1c: 1 cm < tumour < 2 cm in its largest dimension

T2: 2 cm < tumour < 5 cm in its largest dimension

T3: tumour > 5 cm in its largest dimension

T4: tumour of any size extending directly either to the chest wall (a) or to the skin (b)

- T4a: extension to the chest wall excluding the pectoral muscle
- T4b: idema (including orange peel skin) or ulceration of the skin of the breast, or permeation nodules located on the skin of the same breast
- T4c: T4a + T4b
- T4d: inflammatory cancer.

REGIONAL LYMPH NODES **PN**

Nx: invasion of regional lymph nodes cannot be assessed (e.g. already surgically removed or not available for pathological analysis due to lack of evidence).

N0: no regional lymph node involvement on histology and no additional examination for isolated tumour cells

- N0(i-): no regional lymph node involvement on histology, negative immunohistochemical study (IHC)
- N0 (i+): no histological regional lymph node involvement, positive IHC, with cell clusters < 0.2 mm (considered to be without lymph node metastasis)
- N0 (mol-): no regional lymph node invasion histological, molecular biology negative (RT-PCR: reverse transcriptase polymerase Chain reaction)
- N0 (mol+): no histological regional lymph node involvement, positive molecular biology (RT-PCR)

N1mi: micrometastases > 0.2 mm and < 2 mm

N1: invasion of 1 to 3 axillary lymph nodes and/or invasion of MIF lymph nodes detected on sentinel lymph node without clinical signs

- N1a: invasion of 1 to 3 axillary lymph nodes
- N1b: Invasion of MIF lymph nodes detected on sentinel lymph node without clinical signs
- N1c: invasion of 1 to 3 axillary lymph nodes and invasion of MIF lymph nodes detected on sentinel lymph node without clinical signs (pN1a + pN1b)

N2: invasion of 4 to 9 axillary lymph nodes or invasion of suspected homolateral internal mammary lymph nodes, in the absence of axillary lymph node invasion.

- N2a: invasion of 4 to 9 axillary lymph nodes with at least one cell cluster > 2 mm
- N2b: invasion of suspected homolateral internal mammary lymph nodes, in

the absence of axillary lymph node invasion.

N3: invasion of at least 10 axillary nodes or invasion of the subclavicular nodes (level III axillary) or invasion of the suspected homolateral internal mammary nodes with invasion of the axillary nodes or invasion of more than 3 axillary nodes and invasion of the MIF nodes detected on sentinel node without clinical sign or invasion of the homolateral supraclavicular nodes.

- N3a: invasion of at least 10 axillary lymph nodes (with at least one cell cluster > 2 mm) or invasion of sub-clavicular lymph nodes
- N3b: invasion of suspected homolateral internal mammary nodes with invasion of axillary nodes or invasion of more than 3 axillary nodes and invasion of MIF nodes detected on sentinel node without clinical signs
- N3c: invasion of the homolateral supraclavicular lymph nodes.

Distant metastases (M)

- Mx: insufficient information to classify distant metastases
- M0: absence of distant metastases

- Ml: presence of distant metastases

Classification by UICC stage

0 Tis N0 M0

I:T1N0M0

IIA : T0 N1 M0 ; T1 N1 M0 ; T2 N0 M0 ;

IIB : T2 N1 M0 ; T3 N0 M0

IIIA: T0 N2 M0; T1 N2 M0; T2 N2 M0; T3 N1 M0; T3 N2 M0

IIIB: T4 N0 M0; T4 N1 M0; T4 N2 M0

IIIC: All T N3 M0

IV: All T All N M1

HISTOPRONOSTIC GRADING :

There are several ways of establishing histopronostic grades.

The score commonly used is the Scarf-Bloom-Richardson score (SBR grade) modified by Elston and Ellis [72; 73].

This classification applies to all forms of invasive cancer and takes into account three histological criteria rated from 1 to 3: tubulo-glandular differentiation of the tumour, nuclear pleomorphism and mitosis count.

- Tubulo-glandular differentiation is assessed on the basis of the proportion of tubules and glands present in the tumour:

> score 1: well differentiated (more than 75% of tumour surface).

> score 2: moderately differentiated (10-75% of tumour surface).

> score 3: little difference (less than 10% of tumour surface)

- Nuclear pleomorphism: nuclear atypia is judged on the predominant cell population and not on a minority zone.

> Score 1: nuclei that are both regular and less than 2 times the size of normal cell nuclei.

> Score3 : cores :

> The nuclei are regular, but more than 3 times the size of normal cell nuclei.

> Or irregular, with a variation in size ranging from 1 to 3 times that of normal cell nuclei.

> Score 2: everything that is is neither 1 nor 3.

- Mitoses: mitoses must be counted at magnification (400x) in the most mitotic zone and 10 consecutive fields must be counted.

> Score 1: 0 to 6 mitoses per 10 fields.

> Score 2: 7 to 12 mitoses per 10 fields.

> Score 3: more than 12 mitoses per 10 fields.

The total score obtained distinguishes between :

> Grade I: total scores of 3, 4 or 5 (favourable prognosis)

> Grade II: total scores 6 or 7 (average prognosis)

Grade III: total scores 8 or 9 (unfavourable prognosis)

Appendix 3

Information sheet

Identity :

IP: : | |: | |: | | |

Age: | | | (in years) Marital status 1Single 2 Married 3Divorced 4Widowed SE level: 1 High 2 Medium 3 Low

Questioning :

Age of first menstrual period | | (in years) Age of first pregnancy | | (in years)

NP. 3

NP. 3

Exposure to radiation: yes - no - 2 NP- 3 ATCD Family Kc (Mother or sceur or aunt) yes - 1 no - 2 NP- 3 ATCD personal neo: yes - 1 no 2 NP- 3 if yes :

1. contralateral breast 2. ovary 3. colon 4. Other

Reason for hospitalisation

1. Breast nodule 2 - Mastodynia 3 - Breast discharge 4 - Cutaneous sxes 5 - Dep istage

6 - Others...... ... .

Clinical examination :

Inspection:

Asymmetry:

yes.1 no.2

Redness:

yes.1 no.2

You:

yes.1 no.2 Nipple retraction: yes.1 no.2 Nipple discharge: yes.1 no.2

Orange peel:

yes.1 no.2

Palpation:

Number of nodules: | | | Size: | | | | (cm) Siege:

	QSE	QSI	QII	QIE	JQS	JQI	JQE	JQI	Retromam melo na ire
SG									
SD									

Shape : round LI 1 oval |_| 2 irregular |_|3
Other
Outlines : well limits |_| 1 mat limits : | | 2
Consistency : firm |_| 1soft |_| 2
Mobility : movable relative to the pd plane |_| 1movable relative to the supel plane |_| 2
Fixed in relation to the pd |_| 3 plane Fixed in relation to the sup |_| 4 plane
Sensitivity: palnful |_| 1 painless| |2
ADP : yes|| 1 no|_| 0 if yes description :

TNM:T|_JN|_ M|_

PEV: PEV 0 _| PEV1 |_ PEV2 _| PEV3

|_|

Clinical results : NP|

|

Good - **1 Bad - 2 Inconclusive - 3**

Paraclinical examinations:

Mammoqraphy :
MAMMO

Opacity(OP)	- Number: (nodules) (nbr) - Shape: round - 1oval - 2 1obи1ëe^ 3 (frm) - Height: | Ц. **(cm)** (height) - Outlines: circumscribed - 1 indistinct - 2 spicu^s - 3 microlobules - 4masks - 5 (cntr) - Density: high - 1 medium^ 2 low^ 3 greasy - 4 (dens) **QSi QSI QII QIE JQS JQI JQE JQI Retromam metonaire** SG **sD111 1 111 1**
	-morphology: cutaneous.1 vascular - 2 coralliform^ 3 (morph) in rods "4 round^5 with light centre*6 eggshell*7 sëdimentës-8 dystrophic^9 Regular punctiform4 0 suture threads41 powdery< amorphous^la polymorphous ^4 vermiculary.15. -distribution ë-parse / diffuse - 1 regional - 2 segment e - 3 1тëa1re - 4in focus- 5 (distr) ■ **classification** (ACR)
Architectural organisation (DESORG)	Yes - 1No - 2
Asymmetrical density	A concave limits (ACR3) - 1 a convex limits (ACR4) - 2 Mëlangëe has fat (ACR 3) - 3
Associated signs	Skin retraction - 1st nipple retraction - 2 skin thickening 3 stromal thickening 4 Axillary ADP - 5Skin lesion - 6 Other
ACR BIRADS (ACR)	

Ultrasound:

Mass	-number: (nodules) -shape: round.1oval .2 irregular.3 -orientation: paralleled.1 non paralleled -contour: circumscribed.1 non circumscribed.2 hyper echogenic halo.3 -size: |_|| |_(cm) -

	QSE	QSI	QII	QIE	JQS	JQI	JQE	JQI	Retromammary
SG									
SD									

	-echogenic: anechogenic.1isoechogenic .2 Hypoechogenic.3 Hyperechogenic.4 Complex.5 -ombre: attenuation.1reinforcement .2 RAS.3 -effect on neighbouring tissues: compression.1infiltration .2 Oedema.3RAS .4 -Doppler vascularisation: yes.1 no.2 NP.3

	-sx associates:
Other	-Calcifications: yes.1 no.2 if yes, ACR class: -Axillary ADP: yes.1 no.2 -Others:
ACR BI RADS	

Anatomopathological diagnosis:

*Cytology: benign.1 malignant.2 inconclusive .3
*Biopsy: **Tumour** yes.1 no.2
Technique: microbiopsy.1 macrobiopsy.2 extemporaneous.3
Result: Tumour B.1 Tumour M.2 Intermediate tumour.3 Inconclusive.4
Ganglion yes.1no .2
Result: Benin.1Malin . 2Inconclusive.3
Skin yes.1no .2
Result: Benin.1Malin . 2Inconclusive.3
*Operating part: yes.1 no.2
Anapath result:
Histological type:
SBR: I. II. III.
Number of clean-ups: |_||_| (clean-ups)
Number of gg reached: |_||_| (gg)
HR search: yes.1 no.2
Search for RO:
Search for PR:
Vascular emboli:

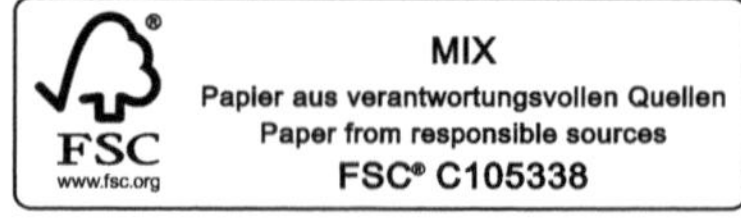

Printed by Books on Demand GmbH, Norderstedt / Germany